Vital Notes for Nurses: Nursing Models, Theories and Practice

Vital Notes for Nurses are indispensable guides for student nurses taking the pre-registration programme in all branches of nursing.

These concise, accessible books assume no prior knowledge. Each book in the series clearly presents the essential facts in context in a user friendly format and provides students and qualified nurses with a thorough understanding of the core topics which inform professional practice.

Published

Vital Notes for Nurses: Psychology
Sue Barker
ISBN: 978-1-4051-5520-5

Vital Notes for Nurses: Accountability
Helen Caulfield
ISBN: 978-1-4051-2279-5

Vital Notes for Nurses: Health Assessment
Edited by Anna Crouch and Clency Meurier
ISBN: 978-1-4051-1458-5

Vital Notes for Nurses: Professional Development, Reflection and Decision-making
Melanie Jasper
ISBN: 978-1-4051-3261-9

Vital Notes for Nurses: Principles of Care
Hilary Lloyd
ISBN: 978-1-4051-4598-5

Vital Notes for Nurses: Nursing Models, Theories and Practice
Hugh P. McKenna and Oliver D. Slevin
ISBN: 978-1-4051-3702-7

Vital Notes for Nurses: Research for Evidence-Based Practice
Robert Newell and Philip Burnard
ISBN: 978-1-4051-2562-8

Vital Notes for Nurses: Promoting Health
Jane Wills
ISBN: 978-1-4051-3999-1

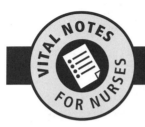

VITAL NOTES FOR NURSES

Nursing Models, Theories and Practice

Hugh P. McKenna
PhD, BSc(Hons), RMN, RGN, RNT, DipN(Lond), AdvDipEd, FRCSI, FEANS, FRCN
Professor and Dean, Faculty of Life & Health Sciences
University of Ulster

Oliver D. Slevin
Lecturer
School of Nursing
University of Ulster

Blackwell
Publishing

This edition first published 2008
© 2008 by Hugh P. McKenna and Oliver D. Slevin

Blackwell Publishing was acquired by John Wiley & Sons in February 2007.
Blackwell's publishing programme has been merged with Wiley's global Scientific,
Technical, and Medical business to form Wiley-Blackwell.

Registered office
John Wiley & Sons Ltd, The Atrium, Southern Gate, Chichester, West Sussex, PO19
8SQ, United Kingdom

Editorial office
9600 Garsington Road, Oxford, OX4 2DQ, United Kingdom

For details of our global editorial offices, for customer services and for information
about how to apply for permission to reuse the copyright material in this book please
see our website at www.wiley.com/wiley-blackwell.

Library of Congress Cataloging-in-Publication Data

McKenna, Hugh P.
Nursing models, theories and practice / Hugh P. McKenna, Oliver D. Slevin.
p. ; cm. – (Vital notes for nurses)
Includes bibliographical references and index.
ISBN-13: 978-1-4051-3702-7 (pbk. : alk. paper)
ISBN-10: 1-4051-3702-9 (pbk. : alk. paper) 1. Nursing models. 2. Nursing–
Philosophy. I. Slevin, Oliver. II. Title. III. Series.
[DNLM: 1. Nursing Theory. WY 86 M478n 2008]
RT84.5.M38 2008
610.7301–dc22
2007039648

A catalogue record for this book is available from the British Library.

Set in 10/12pt Palatino by SNP Best-set Typesetter Ltd., Hong Kong
Printed and bound in Singapore by Markono Print Media Pte Ltd

1   2008

Contents

Preface   ix

1 Introduction: The Case for Theory in Nursing   1
The necessity of theory   1
Theory defined   3
Reflecting on the definition   6
The position so far   9
Do we really need theory?   10
Can we do without theory?   13
Viewing theory in the wider context   16
Final thoughts: our theory for our practice   18

2 Theory from Practice or Practice from Theory?   21
Moving forward   21
The questions begged   23
Next steps   25
The nature of knowledge   34
Theory–practice gaps   46
Science–practice gaps   47
Conclusion   57

3 Knowing and Knowledge: Importance for Nursing   63
Philosophies of knowledge   64
How science develops   71
The move to phenomenology   72
How do nurses know?   74
Categories of knowing   77
Carper's ways of knowing in nursing   79

Linking knowing with theory   82
Research as a basis for knowledge development   83
Developing nursing knowledge through reasoning   85

4   Nursing Theories and Nursing Roles   89
Role theory   90
Interagency/interprofessional changes   92
Confusion surrounding innovative roles   93
Accountability   94
Isolation and burnout   94
Inconsistency in role development   95
Deskilling of generalist practitioners   95
Influence of the medical model on nursing roles   96
Relevance of existing 'grand' nursing theories   100
Relevance of existing 'middle range' nursing theories   102
Relevance of existing practice theories   103

5   Nursing Theories or Nursing Models?   107
Models   107
Theories   109
Classification of theories   113
The metaparadigm   116
Limitations of nursing theories   119
Benefits of nursing theories   122

6   Nursing Theories and Interpersonal Relationships   125
Interpersonal theories of nursing   128
Implications for nurse education   134
Social capital   135
Threats to interpersonal theories and practice   136

7   Selecting a Suitable Theory   141
Problems in selecting a theory   143
Criteria for selecting an appropriate theory   149
Paradigms as a basis for choice   153
Practitioners' values and beliefs as a basis for choice   153
A strategy for choice   154

8   Research-Based Theories or Theory-Based Research?   159
Theory-generating research   164
Theory-testing research   168
Theory-framed research   171
Theory-evaluating research   173
Empirical relationship between theory and research   175
Strategies for theory development through research   178

9   **Evaluating Nursing Theories**   **185**
The words that pave our path   189
Testing and evaluating theory   198
Summative and formative evaluation   207
Evaluation frameworks   211
Conclusion   215

References   **219**

Index   **235**

Preface

This textbook takes you on a journey. It starts by presenting the case for the use of theory in nursing practice. It guides you through the arguments around the extent to which practice influences the development of theory, the definitions of theory and different forms of theory. Insofar as theory is linked to science, the discussion is extended into the relationship between science and practice. The different ways in which nurses know is explored, as is the role of research and reasoning in constructing nursing knowledge.

We describe how new nursing roles and nursing theories have evolved and the importance of middle range and practice theories for guiding practice within these new roles. We tackle with relish the often controversial relationship between theories and models and show how models can lead to the development of theory. We examine these terms in detail and compare and contrast them, taking into account their advantages and disadvantages.

We put forward the argument that nursing is mainly about building and sustaining interpersonal relationships with patients, their families and communities. We outline a number of nursing theories that have interpersonal relations at their core – relationships with patients, families and communities – and the potential barriers to achieving these goals.

We maintain that choosing an inappropriate theory for practice can have damaging effects on patient care. Conversely, we believe that a theory that is appropriate for practice will benefit patients and improve the working practices and morale of nurses. We discuss twelve different criteria that can be used to help you select a nursing theory for practice.

An important part of every clinical nurse's role is to ensure that their practice is informed by the best available evidence. To do this not only must they be practically competent but they must be aware of the importance of theory and research. We examine how theory is generated by research, tested by research and evaluated by research. We also highlight how theory can help frame a research study. We guide you through the process of identifying some interesting occurrences in your practice and how you could develop these into a nursing theory.

Finally, we discuss how the worth of a theory is ascertained. The characteristics of a good theory are reviewed and these are presented as the basis for evaluating any theory. The particular place of testing a theory is considered, and the relationship between theory evaluation and theory testing clarified.

We hope you will enjoy reading this textbook and that it opens up new and interesting perspectives in your thinking and practice.

Hugh P. McKenna
Oliver D. Slevin

Introduction: The Case for Theory in Nursing

'The word praxis is now increasingly used . . . to express a sense related to theory where praxis is practice informed by theory and also, though less emphatically, theory informed by practice, as distinct both from practice uninformed by or unconcerned with theory and from theory which remains theory and is not put to the test of practice.'

Keywords, R. Williams (1983: 317–318)

Outline of content

This chapter covers the following: the case for theory; the argument that all intentional and rational actions, including nursing actions, by definition must have an underlying theory; an initial definition of theory; different patterns of knowing and sources of knowledge; how theory and practice become integrated in nursing *praxis*.

The necessity of theory

Why study theory? What has this got to do with nursing? How can something that is divorced from action, that is by definition abstract and conjectural, be of value to something like nursing that is the most practical of activities? This book will answer these questions. However, it is not an apology for or a defence of theory. Instead, the position adopted from the outset is that *there is no such thing as nursing without theory*. This may seem to be an extreme and indeed audacious claim. Some people argue that in the real world of practice most nurses are not concerned with theory. They know nothing about theory and it is seen as something only of interest to nursing academics. This is perhaps understandable. Many nursing textbooks and journal papers on theory are highly complex, and sometimes seem to exclude the uninitiated by virtue of the obscure jargon used. Yet behind these texts and the views of those who reject them is a reality that is often missed: the fact that every nursing act finds its basis in *some* theory.

The nurse performing such a nursing 'act' may not have a named theory in mind. She may even reject the notion that she *has* a theory that she is applying in this situation. But she does what she does for a reason: she has determined that in this situation she must act in this way. Insofar as there is a reason or purpose in mind, there is a theory. When we are thinking in a rational as opposed to unmindful way (as when we are daydreaming or allowing our mind to wander) we are considering something in an *intentional* manner. We are always seeking to understand, to uncover meaning, to determine how we should act on the basis of our understanding. Later, we will propose more refined definitions of theory. But in simple terms the latter processes describe theorising or *theory construction*. In this sense, theory is not some rarefied academic pursuit. It is something that every nurse is called to do.

Above, we refer to theory construction. From the moment we start to think about something intentionally, we are constructing. What does this mean? When we speak of construction we are referring to how something is built, or how the parts are put together to form a whole. Frequently, we are referring to a building (that which has been constructed) such as a house or a bridge. But when we bring *thoughts* together to form some whole, we are also constructing. In this instance we are producing a *mental* building that also has about it a sense of wholeness, which can be explicated and shared with others through language.

This latter point draws attention to another significant aspect of this process. When we think, we do so in language – a set of symbols that labels the mental images that make up our thoughts and the connections we make between them. Thus a simple phrase such as 'The chicken crosses the road' consists of a number of language symbols (nouns, verbs, prepositions, adverbs, and so on) that express meaning. The fact that our thinking is framed in the symbols of a language does raise a question about how that language may in turn shape *how* we think. This is a matter we return to later in the book. However, what is of importance here is the fact that we *must* use such modes of thinking in our everyday lives. This is necessary not only for attempting to understand the phenomena we confront, but also for determining how we will respond. For example when the above simple phrase is extended to the question 'Why does the chicken cross the road?' we are carried to a different and more complex level of thinking. We seek not only an understanding of the situation, but also possible cause-and-effect reasons for the phenomenon we are observing. And as a consequence of these processes, we arrive at some provisional statement that, while its validity remains to be confirmed, nevertheless suggests to us that if something is done it will result in a specific outcome.

Of course, the dilemma faced by a chicken at a roadside is of little consequence to nurses. But if a question like this is shifted to another context it is an entirely different matter. Thus, questions such as 'Why is the patient crying?' or 'Why has the baby's breathing suddenly become laboured?' are highly important and often life-or-death matters. How the nurse arrives at answers to *these* questions and the actions she takes on the basis of her interpretation of the situation is of highest importance.

We see here that not only does every nurse 'theorise' but also that the quality of the theory that guides her action – for now, we might term this the *soundness* of her theory – is vital. There are issues of how nurses construct theories and issues also of the soundness or utility of the theories so constructed. It might therefore reasonably be argued that such is the importance of theory in nursing that we are obliged, each and every one of us, to address such matters in a constructive way. The aim of this book is to assist the reader in meeting this challenge.

Theory defined

This book is about theory. It can therefore be expected that the issue of what theory actually *is* will be returned to frequently in this and subsequent chapters. However, it is important at this stage to consider at least a provisional early definitive statement on theory. In a sense we have already done this above. There, we suggest that:

> (theory is) thinking in a rational as opposed to unmindful way . . . (in which we are) seeking to understand, to uncover meaning, to determine how we should act on the basis of our understanding.

This is of course a simplification. From a review of statements on the nature of theory in the nursing literature, Slevin defined theory as follows:

> 'Theory is within the cognitive-empirical domain (Chinn and Kramer, 1999). It is the description or explanation of phenomena

and the relationships between such phenomena (Stevens, 1979). In essence, our addressing of such phenomena (those things we observe or are conscious of) leads to the formulation of concepts, i.e. symbolic descriptions of how phenomena cluster or merge into meaningful notions. A theory occurs when these concepts are in turn linked by propositions which state relationships between them (Kim, 1983). Such statements may go beyond the purely descriptive or explanatory levels, to the level of prediction, where the propositions are of such a nature that they state cause-effect relationships between the concepts (Alligood and Marriner Tomey, 2002). In some instances, it is further recognised that theory has a utility value in that it prescribes our actions (Meleis, 1997; 2007).'

Slevin (2003a: 263–264)

It will be clear that the above definition has at its core the view that theory is a construction in the sense that we describe this above. It consists of *concepts* linked by statements that propose particular types of connections that join these concepts together (so we term these statements *propositions*). It can be seen from this that (at least as regards the above definition) for a statement to be accepted as a theory, it must meet the following conditions:

- It must have two or more concepts.
- It must have one or more propositions.
- The proposition(s) must claim a relationship or relationships between the concepts contained in the statement.

Extending our notion of theory as construction, we might view this in terms of a bricks and mortar metaphor as in Figure 1.1. The *concepts* are the bricks. But the bricks may be of different shapes and sizes, and made of different materials. They may be 'people' bricks, 'object' bricks, or even bricks consisting of more abstract concepts such as 'love' or 'justice'. The *connections* between concepts are the mortar. But the mortar may also be of different forms. It may be descriptive, explanatory or predictive mortar. Additional bricks (concepts) may be added, but they must fit the whole – there must be mortar (propositions) that connects them in the process of building (theorising).

Take the question we introduced earlier: 'Why has the baby's breathing suddenly become laboured?' Here we have at least two concepts: baby, and laboured breathing. There may be other concepts hidden around in here, and we may be able to identify these quickly. For example, some object or substance (e.g. mucus – another concept) may be in the baby's air passages (and 'air passage' is yet another concept).

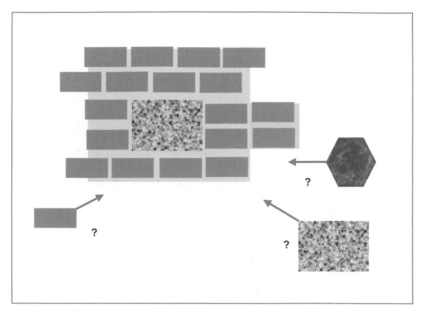

Figure 1.1 Theory as construction.

The baby may be changing colour, rapidly becoming blue (and even 'complexion' of the skin is a concept). To the nurse, these are quickly seen as concepts that are all linked in certain ways. The object (concept) in the airway (concept) is preventing (proposition) the baby (concept) from breathing (concept). This is causing (proposition) the sudden change in complexion (concept) that indicates (proposition) a lack of oxygen (concept). The object or substance (concept) must be removed (proposition) or the baby may end up dead (concept). This may all seem a simplified and indeed nonsensical line of thinking that bears little resemblance to the classical examples of scientific theory, such as the *theory of relativity* or the *theory of diminishing returns*. And of course, the experienced nurse confronted with this situation is not likely to be in any sense going through this sequence of using propositions to relate concepts in a pedestrian and mechanical way. Indeed, she will be doing all this with twinkling rapidity, without even seeming to stop and think. Nevertheless, this rapid theorising-in-action contains all the elements in our definition above.

The definition we propose is a rather complex bringing together of key statements into a composite definition. In one sense it is certainly comprehensive, but in attempting to achieve this it runs the risk of being difficult to understand. It is important therefore to spend some time in reflecting upon the definition and the various terms it uses.

Reflecting on the definition

Theory separate from real-world knowledge and practical considerations

One of the problems we face in defining theory is that it often means different things to different people. For example, we have emphasised in our definition above the notion that theory requires concepts (two or more) linked by propositions (one or more). McKenna (1997) and Fawcett (1999, 2005) drew attention to the fact that some (e.g. Duldt & Griffin 1985; Kerlinger 1986) saw such links as definitive of theory. Others (e.g. Meleis 1997) saw it as sufficient to define theory in a less restrictive way. Thus Barnum (1990) defined theory as that which 'purports to account for or characterise some phenomenon' (p. 1). There is no requirement here to identify concepts and relate them through propositions. Of course, this may not be so far from our definition as it at first seems. If Barnum meant 'phenomenon' to be some state of affairs or happening, if she meant 'characterize' to mean the properties that make up this phenomenon, and if she intended 'account' to mean an explanation of the happening, then she is not too far away at all from the definition we proposed in the previous section of this chapter. Nevertheless, not everyone agrees with this, and in completing Activity 1, you will already be aware that there is no shortage of differing definitions! We must at least be aware that there are these differences, that there are in fact various ways in which people use the term.

Activity 1: Defining theory

Using your learning and library resources, look up the following key terms from the above definition (by Slevin 2003a): cognitive-empirical; phenomena; concepts; propositions; description; explanation; prediction; prescription.

Write brief statements that describe each of the key terms.

Re-read the definition, taking account of the meanings of the key terms included.

Seek out three other definitions of theory through a brief literature search and consider how the above definition compares with these. In particular, identify:

- whether the three definitions omit any of the key elements in the above definition;
- whether there are elements in any of the three definitions that are missing in the above definition, and if you feel this to be a weakness in it.

In one sense, theory is seen as simply a term that differentiates thinking from doing. In this sense the mental muse is often seen to have little to do with the practicalities of the real world. When nurses say theory is of no relevance to their work, it is often this sense of the term they are rejecting. An important extension of this meaning is where 'theory' is used as a synonym for that type of thinking that relates to 'knowing'. Here, theory is in effect the body of knowledge that exists. More precisely, when we speak of a discipline's theory, we are referring to its *body of knowledge*, whether or not this is linked to any practical value.

There is a related sense of the latter meaning, in which theory is held to be separated from and opposed to the real world and our experiencing of it. This holds that theory is concerned exclusively with conjecture and surmise and, as such, has no claim to represent reality at all. One notable example of this was the Italian astronomer Galileo Galilei (1564–1642), who some have suggested was the founder of modern science. Galileo invented the telescope and thus proved that Copernicus (1473–1543) was correct when he proposed that the Earth and other planets revolve around the Sun. This assertion by Galileo was in opposition to the then current 16th-century view that all heavenly bodies revolved around the Earth. This latter position was closely allied to the dominant Catholic Church view of the Earth as the centre of the universe and a central part of God's creation. Galileo's initial thinking was a matter of concern to the church hierarchy. A benevolent pope gave him permission to explore his ideas, but only in a 'hypothetical' way (meaning, in that context, that the ideas would be put forward as a viewpoint and not a claim of proof). When Galileo eventually published his evidence claiming the revolution of the planets around the Sun, he was tried before the Catholic Inquisition, forced to retract, and imprisoned for the remainder of his life. The argument was that in using the concept of empirical *evidence* he was flying in the face of an acceptance of *faith* in seeing the world as God made it. To summon up evidence to dispute faith in God's scheme for the universe was tantamount to heresy. It was not until 1990 (over 350 years later) that Pope John Paul II endorsed a Vatican church commission's finding that Galileo had been wrongly convicted.

This notion of the total divorce of theory from the real world and how we understand it is at the centre of a modern scientific controversy that cuts to the very heart of how science itself is defined. Some see science as containing theory within it as an essential element. Thus:

SCIENCE = THEORY (thinking about reality) **+ RESEARCH** (collecting the data to prove or disprove the theory, or to either support it or place it in question)

But for others, science is a research activity, and theory has no part whatsoever in it. Thus:

> SCIENCE = RESEARCH (the empirical quest for knowledge, whether this is to produce evidence for a truth claim or a less ambitious quest for the best evidence to justify knowledge claims)

and

> THEORY = CONJECTURE (an activity that has nothing to do with science, which produces assertions that are not based upon evidence and have therefore no relevance to genuine knowledge)

The above statements are an oversimplification of how science is viewed and indeed the relationships that exist in respect of science, research, theory and knowledge construction. We return to such matters in subsequent chapters. However, this highlights the view held by some that theory is separate from the real world and our practical knowledge of it.

Activity 2: Introducing the theory–practice gap

The idea that theory is separate from practice is problematic in nursing: if theory has no relevance to practice, it by definition can have no relevance to nursing. Those who reject such a premise nevertheless recognise problems in getting theory into practice. *This is referred to in nursing as 'the theory–practice gap'.*

Do a nursing literature search for this idea. You might find the work by Rolfe (1996) a useful starting point.

Produce a brief one-page (300-word) account of the theory–practice gap. Reflect carefully on your brief account and then re-read the previous section. Finally, consider ways in which this problem of gap may be overcome.

(As this matter is returned to in Chapter 2, you should retain this work in your personal notes.)

Theory aligned to real-world knowledge and practical considerations

In another sense, it is recognised that theory is connected to the real, practical world and is indeed an important aspect of how we live. In this sense, according to Williams:

'(theory is) in effect "a scheme of ideas which explains practice" ... theory in this important sense is always in active relation to practice: an interaction between things done, things observed and (systematic) explanation of these. This allows a necessary distinction between theory and practice, but does not require their opposition.' (Williams 1983: 316–317)

It will be noted that the important aspects of theory are the observation of happenings and the explanation of these. It might be argued that this is an integrated view of theory. It recognises a reflexivity between the empirical (that which is observed) and the explanation or interpretation of this (the theoretical exposition). It in a sense brings together the notions of theory (as thinking) and research (as the act of observing and examining), in effect one interpretation of the term, science, presented earlier.

It is important to note here that this understanding is close to the original meaning of the term, theory. It is derived from the ancient Greek term *theoria*, meaning a spectacle (something that is witnessed). Thus we also have the modern term *theatre*, wherein spectacles are presented on a stage. In ancient Greece it was not possible for everyone to go to some notable event, and of course there were no radios to listen to or television sets on which to observe it! Instead, a *theoros* or spectator was sent to observe the event and then report back. The problem was that the spectator could only report what he saw from his point of view in terms limited by his capacity to interpret and understand. This highlights a vitally important point about theory: it is always a view of the world and what is happening in it from a particular perspective. It can therefore only ever be a partial explanation taken from a particular viewpoint. This is a matter we return to below.

The position so far

We have presented the argument that theory is constantly present and part of our everyday way of living in the world. We are constantly attempting to understand the world or phenomena within it, and how they function. Such rational thinking, whether we call it theorising or use some other term such as problem-solving, is necessary if we are to make day-to-day decisions. Within our own discipline of nursing, even when nurses do not publicly espouse some named theory, on this basis they are nevertheless applying *some* theory or rationale in their nursing work. If this were not the case, if nurses had no theory or rational basis for their actions, this would have serious implications in respect of the safety and wellbeing of their patients.

In carrying the latter argument forward we proposed a definition of theory. This had as its central notion the relating of concepts by propositions that would lead to statements of description, explanation or prediction, and even allow for prescriptive statements about how we *should* act in certain circumstances. However, we also recognised that there are a number of different ways in which people understand this term. We illustrated this by referring to the following alternative viewpoints:

- Theory as something that is opposed to and separate from practice.
- An understanding that sees theory as a body of knowledge.
- A position, close to our own definition, that sees theory as part of science, wherein we formulate statements about phenomena (theories) and then test these empirically (research).
- An opposing view that sees theory as divorced from real science, and relegated to the position of being mere conjecture and having no part in true knowledge construction that must be based on evidence only.
- An argument that sees theory as being aligned to the real world and a means by which we can explain systematically things done and things observed.
- Recognition that theory is always something seen and/or thought about from a particular perspective, and thus by definition a partial and (to some extent) a subjective view of the world or phenomena within it.

It is important that we recognise these different orientations and the views they express about theory. These are matters we will expand upon in the later chapters. However, it is suggested that the general thrust of the arguments we have presented points to the case *for* theory in nursing. To sustain this argument we must determine if in nursing we really do need theory and at a more fundamental level if there is a case for doing without it.

Do we really need theory?

In a novel by Warwick Collins (1992) one of the characters (a Russian police detective) claimed that theory is an essential framing for science. In his work, he always has to have a theory that he will then test in reality through his investigations. If it does not hold, he must search for an alternative theory (explanation) and test this out. The investigation of a homicide can be convoluted and complex, with many false trails. But always it must be carried forward on some basis of a quest for understanding; always, there is the theory, and always it must be tested in the real world. For Collins' homicide detective, theory is clearly indispensable. The issue we explore further here is whether we nurses similarly really *need* theory. The question begged in fact contains within it two issues, one concerning the need for *tested* theory and the other concerning the *production* of theory.

First, do we need a body of *tested* theory that can guide our practice? It might seem that unlike Collins' policeman, in nursing (and health-care in general) the theories we hold must guide our practice, and unsound knowledge can have dire consequences. The argument here runs that (assuming tested theory is defined as the product of 'good' science or research), theory *must* be the basis for our practice. In real-world settings we of course have a name for this: evidence-based practice (EBP) or its many derivative terms (evidence-based nursing, evidence-based medicine, evidence-based healthcare, and so on). We return to the empirical bases of knowledge in the second chapter. However, the condition 'based' hides a danger. It assumes that practice will be unconditionally *based on* empirically derived evidence (tested theory). But in fact, in the real world, all theory (even that tested through research) may at any time be refuted by further investigation, and indeed its application may depend on context. This is why people are now starting to speak in terms of 'evidence-*informed* practice'. The reality is that we are not all that different to Collins' policeman, and his theories can also have dire consequences – miscarriages of justice, execution of the innocent, and so on. We *do*, it might be argued, need a reliable body of knowledge that will guide our practice; and, this knowledge is most valuable when formulated as *tested theory* (state-ments that describe, explain, predict, guide). But we must see this in the sense that 'guide' is a synonym for *pointing the way* rather than *directing* practice.

Second, do we need to produce theory in nursing? Here, it might be noted, we are just like Collins' policeman after all. If we need 'a reliable body of knowledge' this means that in a constantly changing health-care context it must be a *growing* body of knowledge that must be constantly *updated* and *modified*, and always subjected to *tests of refuta-tion*. It may seem that the questions are back-to-front here: surely, if the answer to the first question (Do we need a body of *tested* theory?) is positive, this makes the second question (Do we need to *produce* theory?) redundant! However, the argument here is twofold: as we *do* need the 'tested theory', of course we need to continue to 'produce'. But as such theory is always open to question, and because it is guiding practice in real-world situations (just like with Collins' policeman), we can only use it to assist or inform our practice. We are (as suggested above) always testing the theory in the real situation and each situation is to some extent unique. We have to 'fit' the theory to the situation, adapt it, look for alternatives if it is not found to be applicable, and so on. In so doing we are being questioning, critical, sceptical, constantly analysing, synthesising, seeking patterns in the specific clinical situation, formulating propositional explanations and trying them out. Nurses who do this have been described as 'knowledgeable doers' and some speak of 'intelligent nursing'. Benner et al. (1999) have spoken of 'clinical wisdom'. In our context we might state it thus: the thoughtful, reflective, analytic, insightful, critical practice of nursing is a process of theorising in practice (which we refer to below as *praxis*), and on this basis *every competent nurse is a theorist*. So the answer to the second part of the question becomes: Yes, we need to produce theory (theorise), and that means all of us!

The answer to the second part of our question is therefore that from the cutting edge of nursing research to the immediacy of the patient's bedside we are constantly called to produce theory or theorise. However, we must cast an eye in the direction of those who disagree with us (and also with Collins' policeman!). That is, as we referred to earlier, those who see science as an exclusively empirical activity and as such the only valid source of truth or real knowledge, and who see theory as no more than unscientific conjecture (and not a part of science at all)! Slevin (2003a) has argued against this and takes the view that distinguished scientific commentators such as Popper (1989), Bohm (1998a) and Kuhn (1970) are right in seeing conjecture, tacit knowing and insight, and creative thinking, as essential aspects of science. We return to this point below.

Activity 3: The place of theory in science

Some aspects of theory and theorising we have seen, concern the relationship between theory and science. We have noted that theory can guide scientific activity (research). We have also noted that if a science or discipline takes a particular worldview or adopts a particular paradigm this can influence the type of theory we work with and construct.

Review your literature again, this time looking up the terms science, research, worldview and paradigm. Include the term theory in your search as well. What you should seek are further commentaries on how theory may influence science and how science (or a particular science's worldview) may influence how its practitioners construct and use theory.

Make brief notes for later reference when we expand on some of these issues in Chapter 2.

Can we do without theory?

Thomas Kuhn (1970) argued that science without theory is pre-paradigmatic; that is, haphazard and not science at all. But we must remember that another word for 'paradigm' is 'worldview', a way of viewing the world. If we accept that the quest of science is to discover new knowledge, or truth (and, as we shall see in the next chapter, what we mean by truth is also open to question), how are we to approach any specific paradigm? For example, within the human domain:

- Is the psychological paradigm, or that psychological paradigm currently dominant, the best source of knowledge or truth, as opposed to previous or alternative psychological paradigms, and as opposed to other paradigms, such as the biological paradigm?
- Or, is the biological paradigm, or that biological paradigm currently dominant, the best source of knowledge or truth, as opposed to previous or alternative biological paradigms, and as opposed to psychological paradigms?
- Or, are such paradigms that concentrate on humans as social beings influenced by cultural and social influences the best source of knowledge or truth?

Surely, we might argue that one or other is the best source of truth. Of course, the counter-argument is that none can be a 'best source', that they are in fact looking at different things or the same things from different angles. This relates to one of the earlier understandings of theory we addressed, the idea of theory as a spectacle or view from a particular perspective. The assumption here is that we can divide up the world into such elements as animate/inanimate, organic/inorganic, or (in respect to humans) biological/psychological/sociological, and understand it through the different paradigms or perspectives. The question begged may then be: Do any or all of these accurately describe, explain, or predict the real world or phenomena within it? If we take the view that nursing by definition must look to the needs of the whole person within a whole physical and social world, that its dominant orientation is *holistic*, then devices that fragment the whole are counterproductive. On this argument, theories that are contained within particular scientific paradigms or worldviews (psychological, biological, sociological, and so on), may indeed be something that we can and should do without.

The physicist David Bohm eloquently addresses this issue:

'. . . in scientific research . . . fragmentation is continually being brought about by the almost universal habit of taking the content of our thought for "a description of the world as it is" . . . our thought is regarded as in direct correspondence with objective reality. Since our thought is pervaded with differences and dis-tinctions, it follows that such a habit leads us to look on these as real divisions, so that the world is then seen and experienced as actually broken up into fragments.' (Bohm 1980: 3)

Clearly, one of the things Bohm is drawing attention to here is that a theory is a way of looking at the world. As we noted earlier, it derives from the Greek *theoria* meaning a view or a spectacle. We are in fact looking at the world through particular spectacles or lenses and we can see the world differently if we use different spectacles.

Much of Bohm's work is directly relevant to the discipline of physics. However, the way in which he spoke against the above mechanistic way of viewing the world is also relevant to the human sciences. He used the twin notions of enfoldment and unfoldment (Bohm 1980, 1987). The argument here is that beyond the superficial or mechanistic, there is a meaning enfolded within all things and that our insightful understanding is an unfolding of the meaning that is implicit – he spoke of *the implicate order*, that calls for a consideration of the whole rather than the parts. It is through considering the unbroken whole and its implicit meaning that we move towards the explicit – an under-standing of the entwinement within and between things – their *implicate order*.

In nursing, this recognition of how parts are integral to the whole has been to some extent described by Rosemary Parse (1987) as the holistic 'simultaneity paradigm', as opposed to the particulate 'totality paradigm'. In the former simultaneity position, the person is seen as an irreducible whole, while in the latter totality position, the person is seen as a sum made up of parts. It is also illustrated to an extent by Michael Polanyi's (1966) notion of tacit knowing, a comparison Bohm himself has made. Polanyi highlighted a tacit knowing that cannot be explicated but is implicit in our thoughts and actions; indeed, attempts to explicate can often get in the way of such knowing. It emerges not from empirical trial and error, but from our capacity to see emerging patterns, grasp meanings apparently instantaneously, and arrive at insights. This is relevant in nursing, where we deal not with simple mechanisms but complex persons. Nurses do not work in a factory making mechanical switches – they work in the complex world of human beings where looking at the whole person is preferable to breaking him down into parts such as heart, personality, emotion and so on. Of course, such a suggestion might be viewed as gobbledegook by many dyed-in-the-wool natural scientists.

In the first part of this chapter, a case was made for the value of theory. But it was also recognised that there is the need to keep such theory under constant review (potentially subject to refutation). Kuhn (1970), as we also noted, has argued that a discipline without a body of theory is unscientific. There is an element of common sense in synthesising both arguments. If we *do* need theory that is sound, tested, and up to date, by definition we are speaking of a growing body of theory in the sense that Kuhn proposed. But, in taking this position, we must also be cognisant of the nature of such theory and its limitations. Theories, as we noted above, tend to be specific within a particular paradigm or worldview, and as such provide only a partial view of the real situation (remember, we are viewing the world through a particular lens).

For example, some nursing theories are quite mechanical and break people down into so many activities of living or self-care needs or adaptation modes. Others are more holistic and stress that individuals are not just the sum of their parts but they are more than the sum of their parts. Take the example of a birthday cake with 'happy birthday to Mary' written in icing on top. One way of viewing this cake is to concentrate on the ingredients such as the sugar, butter and flour that it is composed of – a bit like the needs or modes referred to above. Another way is to cut the cake and look at individual slices. After all, the cake is the sum of the slices. But looking at individual slices breaks up the message written on the cake. It could be argued that the cake is more than the sum of its parts. After all it could signify for those present feelings of joy, a rite of passage, happy memories, excitement and so on. So to be reductionist and focus on ingredients or slices misses the whole meaning and significance of the cake.

In nursing, the focus is upon whole persons and the action that takes place between nurses and such persons. The theoretical thinking (and thus theories that may be useful) is by definition drawn from a wider range. Nursing (like so many other applied sciences and areas of professional activity) not only draws from such a wide range, but looks to sources of knowledge that are outside the sciences, and must synthesise all this knowledge to a much greater extent than in a narrower discipline such as quantum physics or behavioural psychology. It becomes clear from this that the answer to the question 'Can we do without theory?' is that in nursing we cannot in fact do without theory. Indeed, we need to draw on a wide range of knowledge that extends well beyond the bounds of theory (i.e. in line with the 'science = theory + research' notion identified earlier). However, we must qualify this by the caveat that all theory is limited in the extent to which it reflects reality. On this basis we again return to one of our earlier premises: we can only view theory in terms of *tentative* descriptions, explanations or predictions. In terms of practice, we use it as a broad guide rather than a specific formula for intervention.

Viewing theory in the wider context

We have taken the view that we cannot do without theory, but that we must recognise on the one hand its limitations and on the other the broad knowledge base that nursing must call upon. This extends beyond knowledge that is propositional and tested empirically (in other words, theory, if we take this to mean a part of scientific endeavour) to other forms of 'knowing'. We need, in effect, to map out, classify, categorise, bring together and organise the total body of nursing knowledge.

One approach is to devise all-encompassing frameworks that show not only the elements that make up the totality of the body of knowledge, but also the relations and differences between these elements. This may be seen as particularly important in nursing, where knowledge is being drawn from many different disciplines and many different paradigms. We call a body of knowledge so structured a *taxonomy* (from the ancient Greek *taxis* meaning arrangement and *nomie* meaning method). Thus, Kerlinger (1986) identified four *ways* of knowing: tenacity, authority, empiricism and apriorism. Similarly, Carper (1978), in the nursing context, speaks of *patterns* of knowing as encompassing: empirics, ethics, personal knowing and aesthetic knowing. We will elaborate upon these taxonomies of knowledge in our next chapter. However, for now we can note that not only is a theory a particular way of 'knowing' from the perspective of a particular worldview or paradigm, but also a construct within a particular orientation (the empirical perspective).

We must remember that the empirical way of knowing is only one of the different forms of knowledge or patterns of knowing. It also has a peculiar property about it, whereby the knowledge gleaned from empirical sources often answers some questions but also creates new ones. This is reflected in the context of theory by Karl Popper when he stated:

'On the scientific level, the tentative adoption of a new conjecture or theory may solve one or two problems. But it invariably opens up many new problems, for a new revolutionary theory functions exactly like a new and powerful sense organ.' (Popper 1994: 4)

and

'[yet] theories are important and indispensable because without them we could not orientate ourselves in the world – we could not live. Even our observations are interpreted with their help.' (Popper 1994: 23)

From Popper's perspective the body of knowledge and how it is organised is not simply cumulative. It is, on the contrary, developing, changing, open-minded, subjected to refinement, constantly being made more robust.

Perhaps we need an additional cautionary reflection here. Popper (1994) was also insightful in criticising the idea of a paradigm or framework, on the grounds that this ties people into a particular way of thinking and – more importantly – particular methodological perspectives. Where this occurs, there is the danger that they not only seek to answer all their questions from this perspective, but in fact attempt to mould the problems to the method they value. He argued that in such circumstances 'a rational and fruitful discussion is impossible unless the participants share a common framework of basic assumptions . . .' (p. 34). As a consequence, those holding to one paradigm devalue the position taken by another (and those in the sciences reject the 'knowledge' of those in other disciplines, and vice versa). This is very similar to the position taken by another 20th-century thinker, Hans Georg Gadamer (1989), who in his work entitled *Truth and Method* criticises the tendency for primacy to be given to method, to the extent that where a particular method or worldview predominates we are only prepared to view reality from that perspective.

All this may lead us to add a proviso to our argument. That is, we should be as critical of frameworks as we are of the theories they categorise and map out. Furthermore, we should endeavour to ensure that *our* frameworks are guides that allow us to explore new perspectives, grow and move forward, rather than being chains that bind and lenses that blind. Because nursing involves caring for whole persons, within whole communities that are contained within wider physical and social worlds, we need the broader view. We need also to be selective in the theories we use, adapting from other disciplines where this works and formulating our own theories where this will not suffice.

Activity 4: The sources of theory

In the latter section we speak of the idea of adapting theories or, if this is not possible, constructing our own theories. This suggests that within nursing there are at least three possibilities: theory 'adopted' from another discipline; theory 'adapted' from another discipline; and theory that is developed in and for nursing.

This is a matter we return to in greater detail in Chapter 2 and later in the book. However, for now, seek out meanings for each of the three possibilities identified above. Write a brief account of each. In each case, list at least three advantages and disadvantages of that theory source.

Final thoughts: our theory for our practice

It is important that in all of this we do not reject theorising. It is essential to assist us in knowing and understanding, and in some instances predicting. But we need also, in our reflections and critical appraisals, to recognise its limitations. In this respect, and in line with our earlier position, Charles Taylor (1995) referred to scientific epistemology as being founded upon knowledge acquisition within a particular perspective, resting for its strength on specific forms of truth claims. Taylor is here using the term epistemology to mean the nature and form of scientific knowledge, and the issue of epistemology is one we expand upon in the next chapter. But importantly, in the context of our current argument, he referred to such *knowledge acquisition* being within a *particular perspective*, with the consequence that its product is of *specific forms*. This is very much in line with the metaphor of theory as a lens through which we view the world. It is also in line with Gadamer's (1989) concerns about 'method'.

The position taken here is not that in nursing we should reject theory because of its potential weakness – the risk that it presents to us a biased and fragmented view of the world. Rather, it is proposed that we recognise the strength of theory and also its weakness. In so doing, we approach theory in a critical manner: making of it robust demands, holding it always open to challenge, recognising that its adaptability to each unique situation is considered. In this respect, Karl Popper's (1999: 14–22) call to *realisation* has informed science and theory. He identified the essential elements of theory thus:

- An explanatory power that is 'an approximation to the truth';
- A 'truth' content that can be subjected to falsification and refutation;
- To be open to the latter processes by a property of 'boldness' that makes transparent claims;
- To have a logical content, that claims rational arguments or consequences;
- To have an empirical content that is observable;
- A narrowing of the gap between idealisation and realisation, or seeking as close to the real world as is possible.

But in this, Popper again and again reminds us that what we are seeing is our interpretation of the real, not the real itself.

Recognition of the fact that we are always witnessing an *interpretation* of reality leaves us in nursing with something of a difficulty. In its original ancient Greek meaning, theory is a spectacle, merely a way of looking at something in the real world. It is not the real world. In this sense, by definition, theory is *speculative*. Yet we are called constantly to 'base' or 'inform' our practice on sound evidence. The questions begged are these: Can we base our nursing practice on the soundest theory, on the best available evidence, if it is always to some degree speculative? How, in effect, do we determine that which is the best theory or soundest knowledge? In this respect, we should of course note that the most reasonable 'call' in this respect is when we are asked to use 'the best *available* evidence'. On this basis, and in specific regard to theory, we must adopt a critical perspective, using criteria such as those identified above by Popper (1999) to establish the viability of the theory.

A further call is therefore to integrate the theory and the practice, a matter we return to in our second chapter. In its ultimate form this is conveyed in the concept of 'praxis' (Williams 1983). Here the idea is that, drawing largely on Hegelian and Marxist thinking, practice must be informed by theory, and theory is in turn informed by practice (see quotation at the start of this chapter). In effect, the word praxis (drawn from the Greek *prassein*: to do) means 'living theory'. Praxis thus understood is knowledge in action. We come close here to thinking of nursing within the current reflective practice discourse and earlier ideas of nursing scholars such as Bevis (1988). Here different questions are begged, such as, for example: How 'practical' is the knowledge? Can the theory be applied in practice?

Such questions have led some (e.g. Dickoff & James 1968; Argyris & Schön 1974) to speak of 'situation-producing theory' or 'theory-of-action', respectively. That is, theory that informs or guides practice. It is such theory that is needed in nursing, and this is of course what we must seek. In this chapter, we have argued that theory is necessary in nursing. We have defined it as a means by which we can describe, explain, predict, or even prescribe how our nursing practice may unfold. But in doing so, we have recognised the problems that exist. There are different views about what theory actually is. There are positions extending from the view that theory is mere conjecture and of no value as a source of knowledge, to the view that it is essential to the construction of knowledge and our application of this in practice. We have, nevertheless, also recognised that theory is always a view from a particular perspective and always a tentative explanation of reality. In so doing, the extent to which it can prescribe or guide theory is open to question. We are, it was argued, always called to challenge the theory, and always called to recognise that it must be adapted to each unique situation.

In one sense this opening chapter has raised a lot of questions about the theory issue. But in doing so, it has arguably met one of its main aims. That is, the recognition that theory *is* an important issue that must be addressed in nursing. In the remaining chapters, we will proceed to address the related issues in greater depth.

Summary

The case for theory was addressed and it was argued that all intentional and rational actions, including nursing actions, by definition must have an underlying theory. Theory was defined, and problems of both loose and specialised meanings were identified. The chapter proceeded to address in more detail the arguments for using theory in nursing, but also the need to recognise the way in which nursing must draw in a practical and pragmatic way from different patterns of knowing or sources of knowledge. It concluded by considering how theory and practice become integrated in nursing *praxis*. The chapter is intended to provide a foundation for proceeding to more detailed consideration of key aspects of nursing theory in subsequent chapters.

Theory from Practice or Practice from Theory?

'Some things are too clear to be understood, and what you think is your understanding of them is only a kind of charm, a kind of incantation in your mind concerning that thing. This is not understanding, it is something you remember . . . We always have to go back to the beginning and make over all the definitions for ourselves again.'

My Argument with the Gestapo, Thomas Merton (1969: 53)

Outline of content

The relationship between theory and practice is explored in depth. The idea that practice is based upon or guided by theory, and the extent to which practice influences the development of theory, are considered. Building upon definitions of theory in the first chapter, different forms of theory are considered. Insofar as theory is linked to science, the discussion is extended into the relationship between science and practice.

Moving forward

This chapter is very different to the first one. In Chapter 1 we were trying to convince you of the importance of theory for nursing. Given that purpose, the case for having theory in nursing was presented in the form of a logical argument. It is hoped that we persuaded you and you are reading on as a consequence. In this chapter, we move to a different level of discourse. We are still considering rational arguments in respect of the nature of theory and its value in nursing. But here, to a far greater extent, we are asking you to be more introspective and to reflect upon certain theoretical and practical issues.

In the opening quotation above, Merton is alluding to assumptions we may make about things. However, when we reflect upon these things, they are not always as transparent and as irrefutable as they first appeared. We have just taken them for granted. Therefore, when we say theory is to do with concepts and the propositions that link them, in a process of extending knowledge about the world, we are making assumptions about a number of things. We make assumptions about what concepts and propositions are. We make assertions about knowledge, but what we mean by knowledge and knowing may be problematic.

This is relevant to you personally. You *do*, as Merton says, need to go back (or at least go into a reflective mode) so that you can make over (review, refine, confirm) your understanding of issues that are vital to your understanding of theory and its relation to your practice. Remember, the title of this book incorporates the phrase *Vital Notes*. We are attempting to present to you in a succinct fashion things that are vital (essential) to nursing theory and its relation to nursing practice and also nursing research. However, the success of this project depends on the vital notes *you* also make, whether these are actual physical written notes, or mental notes that provide you with the grounding to proceed with the issues subsequently addressed.

We claim that the relationship between theory and practice is vitally important in nursing. But within this apparently straightforward statement there lurk a number of potential pitfalls. Not only about what theory actually is and what we mean when we say 'practice', but also about the terms that lie hidden within theory and practice: knowledge, knowing, concepts, propositions, skill, praxis, wisdom, and so on. This is why we are identifying the essentially reflective nature of this chapter at its beginning. It is a call to reflect back to previous positions in respect of theory and practice, not only as presented in Chapter 1 but also what you may have learned about theory previously. It is also a call to reflect inwards about your own assumptions and understandings. However, it may be useful to first undertake the following brief exercise.

Activity 1: Retrospective

Before you proceed, it may be useful to briefly review what we have covered in respect of theory and its relevance to nursing. Continue as follows:

1 Using your internet connection or one in your university/ college, go to the Wikipedia website (you can find it very easily via your search page). Using the search box within Wikipedia, look up the terms 'theory' and 'nursing theory'. (Remember that Wikipedia is an open-source internet encyclopedia that readers can themselves contribute to, so the quality is only as good as the contributors, whose expertise may vary widely.)
2 Review the statements on the nature of theory in Chapter 1.

Compare how theory is defined in Chapter 1 with what is said about theory (and nursing theory) in Wikipedia. Write out your reflections (in no more than 400 words or one A4 page), and if possible discuss with your peers/fellow students and/or teacher.

The questions begged

Our chapter title ('Theory from practice or practice from theory?') begs fundamental questions. Does theory go beyond describing, explaining or predicting our practice? If so, does it inform, advise, guide or even direct or prescribe our 'practice'? Does practice itself provide the most appropriate source of theory for nursing? If theory *does* emerge from practice, what do we do with it after it is mined from the practice situation? Can we assume a reflexive and cyclical relationship between theory and practice, wherein practice is the source of theory, and that theory in turn informs practice? If practice is in some way faulty, what does this mean for the theory derived from it? And, in any case, might it be argued that theory derived from practice in one set of circumstances may not apply well to practice under different circumstances? Apart from theory derived from nursing practice, does theory from other sources (including non-practice sources of theory), or sources that are not theoretical at all, inform nursing practice?

We might go on with such questions, and undoubtedly enter into detailed debate arising from them. Common to all such situations, the questions lead to yet more questions. As we found with our discussion of the opening quotation from Thomas Merton, when we attend to something we find progress hindered because of lack of clarity in respect of things we had taken for granted. All of the questions in the above paragraph depend upon (among other things) how we define 'practice' and how we define 'theory'. These are no small issues. There are many different views about what these terms mean, and sometimes the differences are controversial and hotly disputed. Indeed, just exploring these issues and then proceeding to try to answer the above questions could very easily fill a moderately sized book. We do not have the space here for such deep explorations. In any case, it is not necessary to our purpose, and we will of course return constantly to these matters as we progress through the book. It is sufficient at this stage to recognise that practice and theory may be related in various ways. Figure 2.1 illustrates some possible configurations, and in the remainder of this chapter, the relationship is explored further.

There is one important proviso we should keep in mind. Figure 2.1 emphasises a close relationship between theory and practice, wherein theory informs practice and in turn is informed by that practice. The notion that theory may arise from practice is not new. It has been long recognised within human and social sciences research, in the perspective known as *grounded theory* (Glaser & Strauss 1967; Strauss & Corbin 1998). It is unnecessary for you to follow up on such work now, and we return briefly to this topic in Chapter 6. It is not that such matters may be beyond your capacity to comprehend. Rather, your time is best spent at this point in exploring other dimensions of knowledge and theory.

For now, we can note that the idea is as follows: the theory that will be most useful and most appropriate is that which emerges from the situation being studied (as opposed to theory imported from other situations). In effect, data are not being collected from the situation to test a previously posited theory – the usual approach in research. Instead, by analysing the data, it is claimed that theory will emerge from it (from the ground, so to speak – thus *grounded* theory).

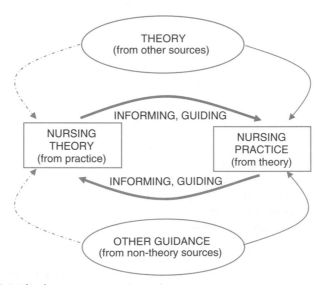

Figure 2.1 The theory–practice relationship.

However, within Figure 2.1, it will be noted that practice is shown to be informed by theory that is practice-grounded, *or* by theory from other sources. Importantly, it is also illustrated that practice may also be informed from other *non-theory* sources.

It would be easy to assume from Figure 2.1 that such other 'non-theory' sources play a minor role in this matter. We speak here of knowledge derived from sources such as the arts – literature, painting, poetry – or ethics, all of which differs from the propositional knowledge characteristic of theory. However, rational as it may seem, some people take the view that theory does not and should not inform practice, and that indeed it has no place in the scientific construction of knowledge (including that constructed to inform practice). From Chapter 1 you will recall that the position in respect of theory is open to dispute, and still fraught with controversy. This is nowhere more so than in nursing, perhaps the most practical of the health and social care professions.

Next steps

Nurses as theorists

We might begin by exploring the position taken by nursing in respect of the questions raised in the previous section, and in particular Figure 2.1. This is no easy task. It assumes nursing (or nurses) may have a shared worldview and a common outlook on issues that impact on the profession and its practice. Unfortunately this is not necessarily the case. Just because nurses seem to be implementing a theory does not mean that they are committed to theory as something important in nursing, or that they themselves are theorising about nursing. Indeed, the extent to which theories *of* nursing, created *by* nurses, that are *for* nursing (i.e. intended to inform nursing practice) are found in the world of nursing practice is open to debate.

As we shall see, there are also issues about using theories (we might term them *imported* or *borrowed* theories) that do not emanate from nursing practice, and indeed may have little support among practising nurses in their day-to-day work. There is always some risk that where attempts are made to adopt such imported unmodified theory in its totality, it will be less amenable to the problems and issues of a nursing practice and consequently less accepted by its practitioners. This is understandable: such theories were initially constructed for another purpose. Indeed, even attempts not simply to *adopt* the theory, but to *adapt* it to nursing are not always successful: at the end of the day bicycles adapted for air travel have always been found wanting in some regards. There is the added danger that by using borrowed theories, nurses will contribute more to the discipline that it was borrowed from than to nursing!

Sometimes (as we noted in Chapter 1), the reality is that theories seem to be largely ignored at the nurse–patient interface. This is problematic. However, equally problematic is the possibility that nurses will extrapolate from this to the position of claiming that *all* theory is irrelevant. In taking such positions, nurses may not even be prepared to acknowledge that their own thinking about nursing – whether this occurs before, during or after practice – can be conceived of as theorising.

As suggested above, such positions may be linked to negative attitudes among nurses towards such theorising. But they may also be linked to a feeling among some nurses that theory is something that is beyond them. This suggests an attitude of acquiescence and resignation among nurses, that they should concentrate on practical issues and leave intellectual pursuits to others. Why might nurses think in this way? There are connotations here about the confidence of nurses as professionals and possibly there are issues of gender: nurses (mainly women) following instructions, with doctors and managers (mainly men) making the decisions (Davies 1995; Slevin 1999, 2003b).

Irrespective of the reasons behind nurses' rejection of theory (or theories), we can see at once that the relationship between practice and theory is at least a matter for debate. However, we must not see this as merely some academic talking shop. If it is important that to some extent sound thinking (let us assume for now that is what theory is) will inform practice, then how nurses themselves *think* about theory, and the resultant *impact* of this thinking upon their practice, is more than a rhetorical question. It is vitally important to the safety, health and wellbeing of those who receive nursing care. Indeed, some would argue that the notion of practice without theory is ludicrous. Nobody would be so uncaring of the health and wellbeing of others as to practise in such a way that actions are carried out mindlessly, without any consideration of the possible consequences.

In arguing that we do actually exist as beings, the French philosopher Rene Descartes made the now famous statement: *Cogito, ergo sum* (a Latin phrase meaning 'I think, therefore I am').

His case was that the very fact that we think and are aware of doing this proves that we exist. In respect of the case being made here concerning nursing, we might turn this statement around: 'we exist (as human beings, and as nurses), therefore we think!' If we accept this premise, then it remains not only to recognise that we think, but to harness this thinking for the benefit of nursing practice and patient care.

An assumption is something that we accept as true. Consider the following assumptions:

- We are active living beings – we *do* things and while some of these things may appear (and indeed are) random and directionless, others are clearly more intentional and purposeful.
- We are rational, thinking beings – this capacity in effect defines our humanness.
- We usually think about what we do or anticipate doing, or have done – thinking and doing are irrevocably linked.
- Such thinking involves seeing challenges or problems, coming up with solutions to these, and reflecting afterwards on the success of such interventions – thus emphasising even more the extent to which the capacity to reflect and evaluate defines our humanness.

One might define the latter processes as theorising. This involves trying to make sense of the world: attempting to describe it, explaining or working out how things 'work' in the world, acting on the basis of such knowledge, on the assumption (which may or may not be proven) that our explanations accurately predict what will happen in certain circumstances.

Activity 2: But monkeys also think!

Sometimes we speak of ourselves as 'human beings'. We noted above the famous Cartesian argument that if we think then we must exist, in order to think in the first place (the term Cartesian refers to the philosopher Descartes). However, to this existence or state of being, we add a human dimension – we say we are *human* beings.

We suggest above that this humanness is characterised by our capacity to think rationally, to solve problems, and to reflect on our strategies or theories in order to evaluate our thoughts and actions. However, psychologists have produced some evidence to demonstrate that animals may also think, and that some apes can even be seen to conduct thought processes that lead to solving problems. Thinking, on this argument, does *not* establish humanness.

Other people suggest that in fact it is not this capacity for rational, reflective thinking that marks our humanness at all. According to some, it is our capacity to make moral judgements (to think and feel ethically), while according to others it is our capacity to respond to beauty (make aesthetic evaluations, which it is argued other animals cannot do).

Continued

It is certainly the case that while other animals may solve simple problems, none have been shown to achieve the level of humans in this respect. Perhaps it is a combination of these different characteristics that make us human. If we are moral beings, we would be called upon to utilise our highly evolved rational thinking to the advantage of others. Theory (thinking about practice) therefore would become a moral imperative.

Reflect upon these ideas. Take some time, and explore your library sources to discern what others say about the property of humanness. When you have done this, reflect further on the above argument – that we are ethically challenged to theorise, and morally charged to arrive at the best possible knowledge to inform our practice.

Nurses as metatheorists

Nurses may also think *about* theory and its importance to nursing and nursing practice. This might be seen (albeit with some degree of tongue-in-cheek) as in fact *theories of or about theories*! A theory *of* theories suggests that we take some position on the nature of theories, their purpose, how we might make practical use of them, and so on. In case you have not noticed it, we are thinking critically about theory and theories and considering their worth or value. That is exactly what *we* have been doing these last few pages!

Such theorising about theory is sometimes termed *metatheory*, a term that usually means a critical appraisal or evaluation of theory. Thus, we might indeed say that the outcome of such a critique would be some understanding (as suggested above, we might term this a theory) about theory. This is itself a highly complex critical activity (McKenna 1997; McEwen & Wills 2007). Clearly, if we are to promote theory, and if it is to be used to inform our practice, it must be evaluated. We return to this topic in some detail later in the book.

Nurses who think critically about theory in nursing tend to be those working in academic or research positions, rather than clinical practitioners. But practitioners may also on occasion reflect upon whether theory is relevant to their practice, and if so what types of theory might be best suited to that purpose. These nurses would not of course use such highfaluting terms as *metatheory* to describe their activity. However, one must recognise that this is done from a position of considerable experience and wisdom. Indeed, nurses often make quite astute judgements about the appropriateness of a theory in respect of its value for informing their practice. In so doing, they are often drawing from years of experience and from a deep understanding of the health-care context.

Levels of theory

Clinical nurses also attempt to analyse practice situations so that their practice is more effective. They do try to think about (or *describe*) the nature of nursing situations, they further attempt to make sense of (or *explain*) what is happening in these situations, and on this basis try to forecast (or *predict*) what would be the outcome of actions they undertake. Based on such predictions they may even stipulate (or *prescribe*) nursing actions. In doing so, clinicians are to some extent mirroring the more substantial theory construction of their nurse scientist and nurse theorist colleagues. However, the ways in which clinical nurses theorise from moment to moment throughout their day, making predictions and prescribing actions, particularly where there is no other theoretical guidance available, is different to formal construction of theory. This does not mean it is unimportant or insignificant. When we think of theory as being of the above different types, we see that – whether on a smaller scale during clinicians' practice, or in more formal theory-construction situations – they are in fact of increasing degrees of sophistication. This is indicated in Figure 2.2.

The increasing levels of sophistication can be noted from Figure 2.2. We must adequately *describe* the concepts within a situation before we can *explain* how these are linked by propositions. Then, in turn, we can only suggest cause–effect or *predictive* relationships when we have such explanations available. Finally, we cannot actually take the risk of advocating or *prescribing* actions until we have firm grounds for claiming predictive relationships. Thus, prescriptive theory is the most sophisticated level of theory that emerges from the development of the three preceding levels.

For a practical discipline like nursing, prescriptive theory is the best that can be had. Nonetheless, compared to established disciplines like medicine, law and divinity, nursing is relatively new. This means that we do not have a large number of prescriptive theories. However, we have an increasing number of descriptive and explanatory theories and in due course these will be developed to become predictive and prescriptive theories.

In Figure 2.2, it can be seen that at the two lower levels, theory simply demonstrates that something is so, and why it is so in terms of propositions that link the defining concepts. At the two higher levels one particular way that concepts are linked (the cause–effect form of linkage or relationship) is the essential factor. Sometimes, the difference between *predictive* and *prescriptive* theory can be unclear. Indeed, sometimes authors seem to say nothing more than that strong predictions will inform practice and in this context are prescriptive theories. On such an argument, prescriptive theory is really no different to predictive theory (other than that we are stating that only well-tested or

PRESCRIPTIVE THEORY
Highest level. Builds upon descriptive,
explanatory and predictive theory. It
recognises the predictive cause–effect
relationships of predictive theory, and
proceeds to **knowledge utilisation** within
specific and contextualised situations. For
example, a decision is made to administer
aspirin to an adult man with a fever and
inflamed joints, and other interventions are
deliberately excluded.

PREDICTIVE THEORY
Higher level. Attempts to predict (forecast
with a degree of confidence) how things work
in the world. The propositions linking the
concepts are now seen as indicating more
specific cause–effect relationships. It is
knowledge confirming, and thus relates to
situations where the propositional links can be
manipulated to show the cause–effect
relationships. For example, administration of
aspirin (acetylsalicylic acid) or paracetamol
(acetaminophen) will reduce temperature in
adults with fever (abnormally elevated body
temperature).

EXPLANATORY THEORY
Intermediate level. Attempts only to explain
why things are as they are in the world. Here
concepts that make up the theory are linked by
propositions that explain the relationships
between them. It is **knowledge building**, e.g.
a solar day for the earth is the time taken for a
single rotation: the earth rotates once in 24
hours; when part of the earth faces the sun, it
is daylight in that part.

DESCRIPTIVE THEORY
Most primitive level. Attempts only to
describe how things are in the world. It is
information presenting, e.g. in daytime the
sun shines, while at night the sun is no longer
visible. Phenomena are classified and
described. An explanation is called for, but not
yet available.

Figure 2.2 The utility of theory in nursing.

'strong' predictive theory should inform our actions). In one sense, this is exactly what prescriptive theory is. Rather than saying (as does predictive theory) the following:

> *if* such an action is taken in these circumstances, *then this will be the outcome . . .*

the prescriptive theory is saying something like:

> *in order that* this outcome will be achieved you must *do the following . . .*

However, to be accepted as having such prescriptive power, prescriptive theory must have gone beyond us merely establishing the cause–effect relationship. We must have considered the evidence for the cause–effect relationship. We must have considered the 'expected utility' of one or some actions as opposed to others. And, we will have taken account of the context. In the example within the prescriptive theory box in Figure 2.2 only the decision (give the patient aspirin) is presented. But behind this, there are a number of other things that have taken place, for example:

- The strong evidence that aspirin *does* reduces temperature is confirmed.
- There is recognition that paracetamol would also reduce temperature, but in some circumstances may be more toxic.
- The fact that while both aspirin and paracetamol will relieve pain equally well (as strong empirical evidence has shown there is no significant difference), aspirin also has anti-inflammatory properties and this person has joint inflammation as well.
- Although aspirin may be contraindicated in some cases (young children, people with bleeding disorders), there is no evidence to exclude its use with this particular person – the theory is taking account of context and the individual case.
- The evidence clearly shows that immersion in chilled water will also reduce temperature (but in this case would be distressing and uncomfortable to the person).
- There is clear evidence that other methods to reduce temperature, such as tepid sponging or using electric fans, do not effectively reduce temperature.

Behind a prescriptive theory, as indicated above, there is a large body of *supporting evidence* (procured through research and systematic review of research findings), and a strong foundation of decision-making that has taken account of *context* and *expected utility*. Importantly, the theory is stated in *prescriptive terms*. In real-world situations, it is presented within treatment protocols or care guidelines. To be so placed it must by definition be *tested* theory, and very well tested indeed. Theory testing is a matter we address later in this book. For now we are noting that a cause–effect theory that is still not well tested can still be termed a *predictive theory*. However, where there is a *prescriptive theory* there is an assumption that one of the essential attributes is that it has already been well tested. Therefore, such theories are not just predicting, they aim to directly influence or determine practice. Thus they are sometimes termed *situation-producing theories* (Dickoff & James 1968; McKenna 1997; Slevin 2003c).

Activity 3: Does theory have a use?

Above we refer to how, in theorising, nurses are describing, explaining, predicting, and perhaps even prescribing. In an important seminal paper, the authors Dickoff and James (1968) described these different theoretical positions (we might see them as theory types) as follows:

- factor-isolating theory, which describes
- factor-relating theory, which explains
- situation-relating theory, which predicts
- situation-producing theory, which prescribes.

They furthermore saw these as progressively more sophisticated theoretical positions. It is not possible to prescribe unless you can predict. It is not possible to predict unless you can explain. Before you explain, you must first describe. Taking it from the opposite direction, unless the basic ideas or building blocks of a theory (we might call them concepts) are sound it will be difficult to explain relationships between them and proceed from this to prediction of causal relationships and prescribing action on this basis.

1   Undertake a brief literature review on the idea of a situation-producing theory and the influence of Dickoff and James's seminal work.
2   Write a brief report of your review. You may find it useful to share and discuss this with your peers/fellow-students.

Theory and practice

In the previous chapter, we attempted to present a case for theory not only being important in nursing, but being indispensable. In carrying this argument forward now, there is some value in reflecting upon:

- the nature of propositional knowledge and the nature of practical knowledge;
- the relationship between theory and practice, the idea of a theory–practice gap, and the linked issue of the relationship between science and practice.

What we are interested in primarily is the value of theory for nursing. Or, more specifically, the utility of theory for practice, and therefore its value in enhancing patient care. There may be other disciplines, such as philosophy or the humanities, where the study of theory may be justified on its own merits irrespective of any practical or utility value, although even this may be debatable. It is hard to visualise that in nursing we would have the luxury or indeed inclination to study theory (even nursing theory) as nothing more than an intellectual exercise. As we noted in Activity 3 above, the argument for theory in nursing rests on the extent to which it has a utility, the extent to which it is a *situation-producing theory* (i.e. one that informs our practice, making it safer and more effective). However, if practice and practical knowledge are distinct from propositional knowledge, the extent to which propositional knowledge is useful in practice is open to question.

Activity 4: Nursing cannot have theories!

In an interesting editorial, Edwards and Liaschenko (2003) presented the following argument (not as their own position, but as one advanced by others):

(a) nursing requires practical knowledge;
(b) practical knowledge is distinct from propositional knowledge;
(c) theories are set out in propositions; therefore,
(d) there cannot be a theory of nursing.

We found in the previous chapter that theory is indeed about propositional knowledge: theory was defined as concepts linked by propositions. But is the argument outlined above convincing?

Continued

> Are practical and propositional types of knowledge different, and
> if so is propositional (theoretical) knowledge to be excluded from
> nursing? Using literature on nursing theory seek out three points
> in favour of and three against the latter position.

The nature of knowledge

Differences: practical and propositional knowledge

A difference is usually made between *practical knowledge* and *propositional knowledge*. This is in fact a notion that is central to the controversy Edwards and Liaschenko (2003) introduced and referred to in Activity 4 above. In Chapter 3, we will be discussing something we term *know-how* as opposed to the *knowing that* form of knowing in greater detail. For now, we can note as follows: *know-how* is a reference to knowing how to *do* something, and it is therefore by definition practical; *knowing that* is a reference to comprehending or understanding something – the concepts within a situation, the propositions claiming to demonstrate links between them – in effect *theoretical* or *propositional* knowledge. Sometimes people also speak of a *knowing of* form of knowledge, which is largely linked with *knowing that* or propositional knowledge, but is limited to simply being aware of the existence of something (we might know *of* a swelling in a human body joint, but we know *that* it is caused by inflammation).

Clearly, while *knowing that* helps us know how things relate and provides useful insights to inform our practice, it is thinking or *contemplative* rather than doing or *practical* activity. It is important to recognise the difference between these two forms of knowledge, the nature of these knowledge forms, and also how such knowledge (practical *or* propositional) comes into being. We should appreciate:

* how these knowledge forms relate to each other; and
* how they impact upon or influence practice.

Practical knowledge

Knowing how

The process of attaining *practical* knowledge is perhaps more difficult than propositional knowledge to explicate. Practical (unlike propositional) knowledge is largely to do with skills acquisition of the form we identify above as *know-how*. It is, as we have noted, recognised as being fundamentally different to propositional or *knowing that* forms of knowing. It is to do with manual skill and the associated psychomotor dexterity, but also extends into something that is more cognitive and indicates an adroitness about what to do in particular circumstances, that is, a form of practical wisdom (Benner 1984; Benner & Wrubel 1989; McKenna 1997).

Such practical knowledge is not easily defined or described in rational language (language that is expressed in terms of logical reasoning, such as 2 + 2 = 4). This is because it is *expressed* in the doing rather than the describing. Sometimes such know-how is termed *tacit knowledge* because it is easier understood as something that resides in the individual, so that the term *personal knowing* is also used (Polanyi 1958, 1967; Slevin & Kirby 2003). The knowledge is resident in this sense because it is the individual (within whom it resides) who knows how to do something. In essence, it is unspoken and indeed cannot be spoken of, except obliquely. It shows itself, quite literally, in the doing.

In this form of knowledge, people can practise an activity until – no matter how complex – it becomes easier to do it at increasing levels of competence. We recognise a smoother and more refined performance of the skills. They become 'second nature', in that the person can perform them without having to think of what is being done in a rational fashion at all. Indeed, the person performing the skill seems to be doing it almost unconsciously, and to an extent, this is so. We start to describe this level of skill as expertise (Benner 1984). However, it is important to recognise that what is happening here is a performance, which is often highly complex and sophisticated.

As we say above, it may seem that this is an unconscious or habitual thing. But that belies what is really going on. Complex patterns and subtle changes are being sensed, and refinements and adjustments are constantly being made without these being thought about in a logical step-by-step fashion. Indeed, to do this would immediately break the rhythm, interrupt the smooth performance, cause the expression of the 'skill' to deteriorate or even collapse in an instant. We might indeed say this is all habitual, that the person is doing it unconsciously. However, do not assume that this is therefore some primitive pattern of behaviour. Modern computers have thus far failed to match the level of sophistication at play here.

Complexity

Just because we realise that propositional knowledge is different to know-how, and that we cannot have propositions that directly guide know-how, does not mean we cannot reflect upon its nature. We can indeed do this, and having a theory *about* know-how is different to having a theory *of* know-how (in the sense of a theory that actually guides it).

Activity 5: Know-how and knowing that

The notion of know-how was introduced by the British philosopher, Gilbert Ryle. His original publication (Ryle 1949) was the first modern statement to suggest that know-how is different to propositional knowledge, and a sophisticated form of knowing in its own right.

The idea of know-how is extremely important in nursing. One interpretation of the position reported in Activity 4 is that nursing knowledge is exclusively of this type. We do not wish to revisit that premise here! However, you may find it useful to revisit the original thinking on know-how.

You should not need to buy or read Ryle's original work. For this exercise, you are being asked to read further around the topic. The internet is replete with descriptions of Ryle's original arguments. Spend an hour exploring these. Then proceed to write (a single A4 page, at most) a case for the importance of Ryle's concepts in nursing.

David Sudnow is a distinguished social scientist. He is also a musician. Note the following excerpt from his description of how his skill as a jazz musician emerged after many years of practice. You should remember that it is in the nature of jazz music that it is an iterative and intuitive process. While there may be (though not always) some thread in terms of a beat and/or melody running through a performance, even the musicians do not know at the start where the music will take them. The piece quite literally moves into new directions, exploring new spaces, from second to second. There is of course a natural end to the piece, but even this is something the musician intuitively senses. Sudnow (2001) wrote of his jazz piano music thus:

> 'I now unselfconsciously follow one piece of advice – heard a long time before from jazz musicians ... *Sing while you're playing*. A "speaking I" is struck by the awesomeness of finding myself singing as I play, singing right along with the movements of my fingers, reaching for next sounds with a synchronous reach of two

body parts, an achievement formerly quite impossible. How do I know what each of these little slices of space will sound like, as a joint knowing of my voice and fingers, going there together, not singing *along* with the fingers, but singing *with* the fingers? How is that possible? I take my fingers to places so deeply mindful of what they will sound like that I can sing these piano pitches *at the same time*, just as I make contact with the terrain.' (Sudnow 2001: 128–129)

This is not something that is exclusive to jazz musicians. Even in the apparently highly structured area of classical music, a notable and famous example of 'singing along' was the celebrated Canadian pianist Glenn Gould. He died prematurely some years ago, but is still regarded by many as the most gifted interpreter of the music of J.S. Bach, and Gould's two recordings of Bach's *Goldberg Variations* (made almost 30 years apart) are considered to be perhaps the definitive piano recordings in the classical music genre. In most of his recordings, despite the attempts of sound engineers to suppress it, Gould can be heard humming. He is in a world in which voice and fingers are complementing each other, but where the artistry is directed into sound through fingers.

What makes David Sudnow's account so fascinating is the extent to which he approximates something close to describing exactly what is going on in a complex skill. But it is only an approximation. He does not *really* understand it himself; or, at least he does not understand it in rational terms that can be explained in logical language. He does of course *know* in certain ways. He knows how to perform this complex skill (jazz music performance), something that we have referred to as 'knowing how' or know-how.

This knowing is also an awareness, and indeed a highly honed and sensitive awareness within which the performer knows the next step (in Sudnow's case the next sequence of keys) without knowing *how* they know this. Sudnow, who has explored this phenomenon in depth, and written a book about it, can only speak about the 'awesomeness' of this, saying 'How is that possible?' The famous expression of Michael Polanyi (1967) that 'we can know more than we can tell' is clearly at play here. Sudnow is one of the most prominent social scientists in the United States, indeed the whole world. He is a communicator *par excellence* and in his book has presented a widely acclaimed account of such knowledge in action. Yet, in the end, Sudnow can only attempt to explain such forms of tacit knowing up to a certain extent. Rational explanations can take us no further.

It is not only that the practical knowledge being exhibited is by definition complex. It is also because the language of description, which is the language of propositional knowledge, theory and rational thinking,

Activity 6: 'We can know more than we can tell'

Note how the juggler uses first two balls, then three balls, then four – all apparently identical. They spin through the air, each in their own trajectory. Imperfections in their shape, slight variations in weight, air currents in the immediate vicinity – all these variables and indeed others cause each ball to behave differently. But the juggling goes on – smoothly, without interruption, and we are dazzled by the perfection of shape and motion. But ask the juggler (during his act) to take account of all these 'variables' that are affecting the balls. In an instant, the smooth co-ordinated motion of spheres will become disjointed and irregular. Soon balls will start tumbling to the ground. Indeed, after a performance, ask the juggler what factors he had taken account of, and how he kept the balls in motion, and he will be nonplussed. We will get an answer something like 'Well, I just did it.' It is not that in the act of juggling the juggler was in some subdued state of awareness. Indeed the very opposite is the case. There is something highly complex going on here that demands and indeed exists as a heightened state of awareness of the activity. It is a doing or performing activity not easily expressed in rational terms. In a sense there are – quite literally – no words to describe it.

Reading
Briefly look up references to Michael Polanyi and his ideas about tacit knowing and personal knowing. You may recall we introduced his work very briefly in Chapter 1. Particularly useful is his famous phrase 'we can know more than we can tell' – a phrase he used in attempting to explain why people find it difficult to describe such things as skills. Also look up the work of American nurse Patricia Benner, particularly her work on clinical wisdom and expertise.

Reflection
Try in your own words to explain the nature of such complex practical knowledge. It is best to try writing this (in about one A4 page or 400 words), as this challenges you to clearly state your thoughts.

Action
Then, if you have an opportunity, and you are in the clinical area, observe an experienced nurse undertaking a complex nursing activity. Then ask her: How did you do that? Does she also know more than she can tell?

is not suited to uncovering what is going on. Terms such as personal knowing, tacit awareness, intuitive responding are in fact almost alien to this scientific language.

Practical knowledge as performance

Practical knowing, as noted above, is largely a performative knowing. That is, it is a performance art or an expressive art form or skill, in that it exists exclusively within the act of doing. As may be clear from the discussions above, it is difficult to express in words, and when we try to do so it is already in the past. In a sense, it is already gone and beyond our grasp.

It is possible that such know-how knowledge is less valued than know-that knowledge. Students often look with astonishment at experienced nurses who are performing a highly skilled task. The aesthetically pleasing art of the doing – almost without thinking – is perceived by the student to be extraordinary and they think they will never be as skilled. The nurse probably thinks it is ordinary and one day when qualified and experienced the student too will perceive it as ordinary.

We will return to the possibility of reflecting *during* practice later. That is, the process of contemplating what we are doing as we are doing it. Such a notion is difficult not only because by the time we do something it is already in the past but also – as suggested earlier – attempting to think about the practice *as* we do it may (as in the example of the juggler) lead to a deterioration in performance. However, the suggestion that at least some aspects of practice are beyond our cognitive grasp (in terms of rational explanations) is a rather astounding realisation in respect of nursing, or indeed in any healthcare profession. We are saying, in effect, that a substantial amount of nursing activity is beyond our capacity to describe in rational or propositional terms. It is beyond theory! Furthermore, because it can only be expressed in the doing it is also to some extent beyond the capacity of evidence-based healthcare. If the arguments presented here hold, there are important aspects of practice that are not amenable to evidence as they cannot be addressed in evidential (propositional) terms at all! They may be referred to as 'practice-based evidence' rather than 'evidence-based practice'!

Practical knowledge as sophisticated knowledge

While the examples used earlier are from areas such as music and juggling, the principles underlying such forms of knowing are similar in all practice-knowing situations. This may seem a rather exotic claim to be making in respect of nursing. However, some of the skills involved in nursing require every bit as much in terms of dexterity and coordination of mind and body as does an activity such as juggling. And in nursing we also find that our practice is every bit as creative as the jazz performances described by David Sudnow (2001), and involve the need to respond appropriately to often instantaneous and chaotic changes in circumstances.

In an interesting paper, Max van Manen (1999) differentiated between what he terms *gnostic* and *pathic* touch. In gnostic touch, the clinician is touching, feeling (palpating) to obtain knowledge. In this sense he is not touching the other in a personal or relational sense. He is in an almost mechanical sense trying to feel through, in order to gain this knowledge (is there a swelling, what degree of tenderness exists, are the anatomical structures normally aligned?). He is feeling through the *body*, not touching the *person*. Thus we have the term diagnosis (from the Greek terms *dia* meaning distinguishing, looking through, to discern + *gnosis* meaning to know, knowledge). The *pathic* touch, conversely, is a touching of or reaching out to the person. From its Greek origins of *pathos* meaning suffering or hurt, we find that pathic touch reaches out to comfort, to relieve pain.

There is a great deal of skill involved in these touches. The diagnostic touch is only acquired through extensive experience and a building up of expertise. There comes a time when the expert doctor or nurse diagnostician's powers (certainly in respect of the diagnostic touch or palpation) appear almost magical. They are every bit as astounding and awe-inspiring as Sudnow's jazz riffs. This is also so of the pathic touch that involves a reaching out not to the physical body, but to the person in a healing purpose. This may involve highly developed skills of massage or manipulation. But sometimes no less effective is the touch that conveys the way in which the nurse is simply present, there *for* the person, reaching out to their pain and aloneness. We speak here of knowing when to reach out, whether to do so in silence or with voice as well as touch, the knowing how to listen, the knowing what to say or not, in each given moment.

All these are sophisticated skills that extend beyond psychomotor actions, often requiring responses that differ from encounter to encounter, and often even within each encounter. But perhaps what van Manen's work also shows is how what we have called practical knowledge and what is termed theoretical or propositional knowledge come together in practice. In both the gnostic and pathic touch, there are tacit dimensions of knowing of the form discussed earlier. However, there is also a recognised need to integrate this with propositional knowledge, The diagnostic clinician (doctor or nurse) is using a highly developed skill of palpation, but he or she must relate this to knowledge of the anatomy, physiology and pathological processes of disease. Similarly, behind pathic touch, and the practical knowing of how and when to use this, is a high level of knowledge derived from the human and social sciences, and from the humanities. In these examples we come to a simple but nonetheless profound realisation.

While practical/know-how and theoretical/knowing-that knowledge forms are very different, they share one vitally important characteristic. They are both focused upon the practice of nursing. They both contribute to safe and efficient treatment and care in respect of health and wellbeing. And, importantly, they are not opposed or disruptive to each other, but of necessity complementary. We need to know *what* to do (theoretical propositional knowledge), and we need to know *how* to do it (practical know-how). In delivering adequate nursing care, one without the other will not do.

Activity 7: From pathic to sympathetic

Words commonly used in clinical practice (and indeed in other areas concerning human relations) are *empathy* and *sympathy*. These are derived from the Greek *pathos*. You may recall this term connotes feelings or emotions, often extended to include feelings of suffering.

The terms sympathy and empathy, while derived from the same etymology (*pathos*) are said to be different modes of relating to others.

Do a literature search for these two terms. Consider how each may contribute in practice situations. There is no further reading or writing work to be done here. However, over the few days after reading this, attempt to identify what you feel are examples of sympathy and empathy being acted out in your world. To what extent are these examples accompanied by what we earlier termed pathic touch?

Propositional knowledge

Rational knowing

We shall be considering propositional or theoretical knowledge in more detail in the next chapter. We also introduced some ideas about this in Chapter 1, particularly in respect of the empirical sources of such knowledge. However, it is necessary to address some ideas about this here, as an essential aspect of exploring the theory–practice relationship. In one sense, this is easier than describing what we term practical knowledge above. Through being based upon reasoning and intentional thought processes, propositional knowledge is perhaps more easily expressed in the same rational terms. This is best understood if we recognise that a *proposition* is in essence an *idea* rather than a *thing* (some object that exists in the real world) or an *action* (some practical deed). More specifically, it is an assertion that something exists or that some relationship or other applies. Implicitly, this means that the proposer (the individual or individuals making a proposition) believes or assumes the existence of the relationship in question. But the assertion is still *in question*. That is, it still has to be shown and in this sense it is open to question until it is adequately demonstrated. This is very different to practical knowledge which is not an idea being asserted, but is demonstrated only in action – we know how to *do* something, or we do not, as the case may be. Propositional knowledge can be seen as emerging in two quite different ways.

A *priori* propositional knowledge

Here knowledge is taken as arising *before* experience or, perhaps more accurately, without the necessity of experience. It is termed *a priori* to denote that it precedes experience or the need for this. Knowledge of this form is said to be independent of any need for supporting evidence or experience. It is, as is often said, self-evident. Its truth or its character of trueness is quite literally contained within it. While it is tacitly recognised, it is still taken as propositional insofar as it is deemed rational and reasonable to hold the knowledge as true or acceptable. We can for example propose that $3 + 3 = 6$. We can see that if there are three oranges sitting on the table and another three beside them, there are six in total. We do not need to call on prior experience to know this, we know it already – and we do not even have to see the oranges on the table to work it out.

A *posteriori* propositional knowledge

Here knowledge emerges *from* experience, and we make deductions arising from this. In this instance, it is termed *a posteriori* to denote that it is derived from empirical experience which in all instances precedes it and is its source. This is not necessarily limited to experience of the external senses (sight, sound, smell and so on), but can include experiences of memory and introspective experience (the experience of previous thinking about or reflection upon the subject). Knowledge of this form is what people usually mean when they speak of *scientific* knowledge – knowledge based on evidence that is derived through research.

Justified knowledge

We state above that the nature of knowledge derived by *a priori* or *a posteriori* means is that it is something held to be true or acceptable. However, the conditions necessary for knowledge to be acceptable usually involves how it meets the test of being *justified true belief.* This is widely held as the test of knowledge. First, we must believe something is true. Second, we must have a good grounds for holding this belief: it must be justified on the basis of rational logical thinking as in *a priori* knowledge, or on the basis of observable evidence as in *a posteriori* knowledge. Third, it must be true. It is possible to believe something is true, to have what appear to be strong justifications for the belief, but for the knowledge to be false rather than true. Conversely, we may assert that something is true, have no really good grounds for justifying the belief, but yet by good luck or chance it is true. Philosophers who study knowledge would argue that, even if the knowledge is true by chance in the second case, in both these examples, the knowledge is not considered to be sound knowledge.

However, we must be careful of giving an impression that this all relates to the idea that there can be absolute truth. Truth (or more properly accepted knowledge) is a relative thing. It is very much embedded in context and culture, and is furthermore held to be always open to critical review – indeed this is taken to be its strongest point! Therefore, to the above three conditions (belief, truth value and justification) we add here a fourth condition – *defeasibility* (which in this context is taken as a potential or capacity to be defeated). That is, such knowledge is always by definition *propositional*, and that is exactly why we use the term. Propositional knowledge is always conditional: we recognise that at some future time it may be shown to be inaccurate. Indeed, nowadays we do not usually judge knowledge on the idea of truth at all. We judge it on the extent to which it withstands challenges. Later in the book we will again be looking at the work of the scientist and philosopher Karl Popper. In his book, *Conjectures and Refutations*, first published in 1963, he argued that knowledge should be judged by the extent to which proposed knowledge (conjecture) can withstand attempts to reject it (refutation).

Propositional knowledge as theory

Knowledge, once constructed, must be packaged and presented. The presentation of knowledge we speak of here is in fact theory: theory is a statement about a piece of knowledge. As we noted earlier, it may just describe something; it may explain how the thing is – with propositions that link its constituent concepts; it may go further to demonstrate how these linking propositions show cause-and-effect relationships, thus allowing us to predict; where our predictions reach certain levels of predictive strength and reliability, we may use them to prescribe. As we noted in Figure 2.2 earlier, theories having increasing levels of sophistication, from descriptive theory up to prescriptive theory.

In some instances, it is not so much theory that is specific and explicates operational research findings (by explaining, predicting, and so on) that causes controversy. It is rather the more abstract theoretical statements. Later in the book we will be returning to such theoretical entities or types. These are often termed (in increasing levels of abstraction):

- *Micro theory and hypotheses*: theory that is expressed in concrete and researchable terms, and very specific to a knowledge issue. This is sometimes referred to as practice theory.
- *Middle range theory*: theory that is still expressed in terms that are sufficiently linked to the specific setting so as to at least allow for testable hypotheses or research goals to be stated. Such theories are broad enough to retain a view of the discipline and its general progression, yet specific enough to identify the empirical work that will advance this progress.
- *Macro theory or grand theory*: very abstract statements covering issues at a level of abstraction not amenable to research testing. Thus, theories about nursing (as a profession) *are not intended* to be reducible to testable hypotheses. They are intended to provide worldviews, to help us map out our discipline's areas of activity, give general future direction, and so on. Such grand theory is too abstract to be restated and/or tested in empirical terms.

Some people also add a fourth form at the most abstract level (above grand theory) that they term metatheory (McEwen & Wills 2007). In fact we discussed metatheory separately earlier in this chapter (taking the view that metatheory is *about* theory, rather than being itself a *form* of theory). Others speak of two theory types – grand theory and middle range theory. According to Fawcett (2005), middle range theories are specific enough to allow empirical *indicators* to be drawn from them.

These empirical indicators – which are by definition concrete and specific – allow data to be collected and tested (thus validating the (middle range) theory. Fawcett does not see these indicators as theories, but they fill that space containing what others define as practice theory, micro theory or hypothesis.

All this may be a little confusing to you. We speak of theory as being of different levels of sophistication (descriptive, explanatory, predictive, prescriptive), and also of different levels of abstraction (hypothesis, middle range theory, grand theory). And even in the latter case we find that some speak of four levels of abstraction (adding the fourth theory type *metatheory*), while others speak of only two levels (middle range theory and grand theory). Perhaps Fawcett (2005) presented the easiest way of thinking of theory: grand theory provides broad direction to the discipline; middle range theory provides testable hypotheses for operational practice (as outlined in Figure 2.3).

In a later chapter we consider how theory is analysed, evaluated and tested in more detail. However, Figure 2.3 indicates the processes that are involved in respect of testing theories that will be used in making critical decisions about practice interventions. It also serves to illustrate important aspects of the theory–practice relationship.

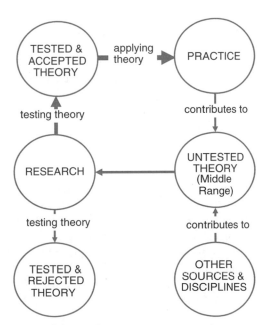

Figure 2.3 Propositional theory: from conception to application.

Theory–practice gaps

The idea of praxis, discussed in Chapter 1, allows for no separation and indeed no distinction between theory and practice. The argument was that practice is by definition informed by some theory, that indeed praxis is a form of practice that we might term *living* theory: good practice is good theory in action. However, some see practice and theory as separate and discrete entities and some view the two concepts as not only separate but also discordant ideas. Even in those instances where it is argued that theory and practice are in fact complementary, it is recognised that there is a challenge to be faced in bringing theory and practice together.

This separation – between theory and practice – is a matter frequently debated in nursing and indeed other professional contexts (Rolfe 1996; Slevin 2003c). So much so, that the term theory–practice gap has become almost shorthand for referring to the whole debate surrounding theory and the difficulties people have experienced in bringing theory into practice. For some, this is not a matter for concern: not only are the two terms separate, but desirably so. This, it may be recalled, is a view sometimes expressed by those who see nursing as practical and not involving theory. It is also a view held by those who see theory as largely conjecture and not a valid aspect of science, arguing instead that practice must be based upon the best scientific *empirical* evidence. However, for others, theory is viewed as essential. It is the basis of science, and theory tested through research is seen to be the basis of best practice. Here, any separation of practice from theory is seen as problematic.

As we noted in the previous chapter, there are a number of explanations about why the gap occurs, why theory is not used in practice. We noted, for example:

- a failure on the part of educators to adequately convince practitioners of the value of theory and/or to adequately prepare them for using such theory;
- ineffective change in management infrastructures and strategies for introducing innovations, including theory;
- negativism on the part of staff (often extending beyond theory to any other change or innovation) – whether or not such negativism is to a greater or lesser extent understandable for various reasons;
- recognition by practitioners that theory being promoted from above is sometimes inappropriate and ineffective – as adopted (unchanged) theory borrowed from other sources, or as adapted (changed or refined) theory.

The issue in Activity 4 earlier in this chapter raises an additional and perhaps more serious reason for the gap:

• given that theory as propositional knowledge and practice knowledge (sometimes termed 'know-how') are entirely different forms of knowing, there will always be a gap – it is as inappropriate to try mixing them together as it is to try mixing oil and water. Of course, as we suggest earlier, that is not to say that the two forms cannot and do not complement each other. Indeed it was suggested then and is now emphasised once again: we need to know *what* to do and *how* to do it, and one without the other will not do.

Activity 8: Different ways of knowing

Practical knowledge is: knowing-how, contained in the doing, tacit, intuitive, personal, complex, performative. Propositional/theoretical knowledge is: know that, descriptive, explanatory, predictive, prescriptive, contemplative, rational, justified.

   The above are some of the differences suggested between these two forms of knowing. Make a two-column table and using library searches make two comprehensive lists of the characteristics that differentiate the two types of knowing. Use these lists to construct your own brief (150-word) statement defining each type. Keep your written work on this assignment for referring back to – particularly when these issues are revisited in Chapter 3.

   The important issue in all of this is as follows. Insofar as theory to some extent enhances practice, and insofar as the practice situation is a testing field for theory, wherein it can be both tried and refined, any gap between the two is potentially problematic. While we can accept that practical knowledge or *know-how* is different to theoretical or *know-that* forms of knowledge, we must also accept that the latter has a part to play in guiding our rational actions. Finally, there may be issues in respect of how science is linked to the real or practical world, particularly where theory is seen as a part of science.

Science–practice gaps

Science and reality

An interesting extension of the theory–practice gap theme is as follows: the activity of producing propositional knowledge (that is, scientific knowledge) is sometimes also viewed as having no necessary link with the real world. Therefore, insofar as theory is a part of this scientific enterprise, it too is held to be dissociated from reality. Such thinking rests on the assumption that theory is essentially an element of science. The image of science as divorced from the real world or reality conjures up the fictional images of the unworldly scientist, the person who lives in a world of ideas rather than reality. This is also where we get fictional notions such as the 'absent-minded professor' who is so busy solving an abstract problem that he has forgotten to put his trousers on! While such caricatures may not exist, there is an element of truth to the suggestion that scientists may indeed become separated from the real world, to the extent that they cease to take an interest in anything outside the laboratory. The unworldly researcher, the mad scientist, the absent-minded professor and the unreal and dreamy world of academia within its ivory towers are all well-known images. It is sometimes such images that lead very practical people like nurses to discount science, and theory, as being of little relevance to the real world.

Of course, this depends on what we mean by 'the real world'. In a narrow or technical sense *reality*, as a psychological or philosophical concept, brings into question the actual *existence* and nature of an object as opposed to the *appearance* (to us) of the phenomenon. As illustrated in Figure 2.4, how an object appears to us may approximate reality to some extent, but it never actually equates to it. The thing that exists

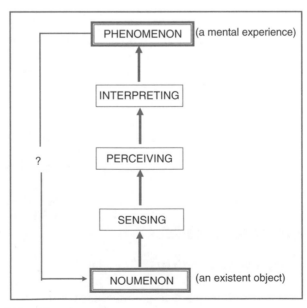

Figure 2.4 The thing observed.

out there (the *noumenon*) is different to how we experience it through our senses (the *phenomenon*).

Indeed, these ideas, when taken to their extreme, can be found in the orientations within philosophy known as idealism and realism. The term *idealism* has been used to describe the position that reality does not exist outside of ideas. Taken to its extreme, it is some elaborate mental construction and there is in fact no physical world out there at all. In other words, we and our total world are thoughts or ideas in the mind of some being (the nature of which may be God or some other cosmic being). The alternative view entitled *realism* argues that there is indeed a real physical world out there. According to this argument, the fact that different individuals perceive the same thing confirms that it must exist. The counterargument of the idealists is that even the people who are doing the perceiving are part of the ideational construction!

Such rather abstract deliberations may be of little interest to you at this stage in your studies. However, you should nevertheless take seriously the need to be sceptical about the information presented to you. While it may be unreasonable (or at least unprofitable) to question seriously the existence of the world we are observing, we should nevertheless be guarded in assuming that what we are observing is reality exactly as it is. It is something of a paradox that on the one hand science (and scientists as researchers and theorists) is devalued for not being in touch with the real world, when in fact that so-called 'real world' is itself open to question. This situation is even more astonishing when we realise that we need this very same science to help us view the world critically and objectively!

Science (and theory) divorced from concerns about the use of science and technology

If science is seen as having nothing to do with everyday life, or what happens in the real world (i.e. is concerned with knowledge construction, not its practical application), we are creating yet more distance between theory and practice. In the past, scientists took the position that they were in the business of discovering knowledge, of establishing what was true in respect of things or phenomena observed in the world. What people did with this knowledge, so the argument ran, had nothing to do with science. For example, splitting the atom was a great scientific achievement; the fact that it led to many deaths (see below) may be considered as not the fault of scientists.

In effect, scientists recognised only a moral or ethical responsibility in respect of the *authenticity* of their work, not for any *consequences* emerging from it. That is, they accepted responsibility to adhere only to certain principles of research ethics. In this respect, the dominant moral obligation recognised was that of absolute truthfulness in conducting research and reporting findings. Other ethical principles recognised in science today (e.g. as derived from the biomedical ethics of Beauchamp & Childress 2001) relate to ethical principles such as beneficence (doing good), non-maleficence (doing no harm), autonomy (respecting the right to choose or give informed consent) and justice (equality and fairness – other than that aspect of justice pertaining to truthfulness). These were often largely ignored, even in respect of issues such as seeking full informed consent from subjects being studied. Indeed, in some instances the wellbeing of subjects being researched (humans as well as animals) was blatantly ignored or even knowingly compromised.

Such positions have been characterised in literature in the frequently portrayed ruthless and often 'mad' scientist, perhaps most notably in Mary Shelley's *Frankenstein* (1996/1831) or in Stevenson's (2000/1886) Jekyll and Hyde characters. However, modern-day literature is equally if not more frightening in its accounts of immoral science, such as in John le Carré's (2001) *The Constant Gardener*. This is a story of the exploitation of poor countries by multinational pharmaceutical companies practising unsafe and unethical science in the developing world. In this work, so characteristic of le Carré's books, there is a well-researched plot, so that what is happening in the fictional account reflects fairly accurately the worst of the real-world dark side of international pharmaceutics. Here, the issue is not merely that of unawareness of the real world or of other people, animals and the environment in general, on the lines discussed in the previous section. In this instance, there is an actual *lack of concern* that begins to beg serious ethical questions.

Activity 9: Science in the clinic

We have considered how science may not be fully attuned to the real or practical world within which we live, and also how science may recognise no moral obligation in respect of this world. It was even suggested that science might blatantly further its own interest at the expense of others.

We do need research to provide the knowledge needed for advancing medicine and combating disease. This, so it is argued, makes it necessary to test treatments and drugs on animals and eventually on people. There are risks that in such activities there may be inadequate attention given to the welfare of those involved. This is increasingly recognised within the National Health Service and research institutions, particularly where responsibilities in respect of 'research governance' are addressed.

Look up the terms research governance and clinical trial. Consider how these areas may impact upon nurses' responsibilities in respect of the safety and care of their patients. You may elect to make some notes, but you are only being asked to reflect on these issues.

Science (and theory) failing, or saving, the world

The limited concern of science for moral issues really changed with the advent of nuclear physics, particularly at the end of World War Two, when this extended into the development of nuclear armaments. Scientists increasingly acknowledged that they had a responsibility to be mindful of the consequences of their work. Indeed, some of the scientists involved in the Manhattan Project at Los Alamos in the USA never recovered from their intense distress and guilt at the devastation wreaked by the two atomic bombs they had invented being dropped upon Hiroshima and Nagasaki. The argument was often advanced that the use of these devastating bombs, which led to the deaths of hundreds of thousands, was justified as this act shortened the war and saved millions of lives – Japanese as well as American, European and others. However, at a time when the war was coming to an end and Japan had already raised the possibility of negotiating peace, this was of little comfort to those who had designed these devices and then were having moral qualms.

It might indeed be suggested that from the end of World War Two, at mid 20th century, science acquired a conscience. The emergence of an ethics of science certainly goes back earlier than the 1950s, but from that decade it reached a new level of importance. Not only did science acknowledge its impact upon the world (and upon humanity) but it also (to a greater or lesser extent) embraced a moral obligation to attend to that possibility. Of course, here also it must be recognised that there are variations not only in terms of degrees of moral obligation but also in terms of the nature of that obligation.

To some extent the modern scientific community has become aligned in two opposing camps. On one side a largely 'green' and populist grouping is concerned with ensuring that science does not harm our environment and also that its discoveries are geared toward ecological protection and benefiting society in general. On the other side a largely opportunist and capitalist grouping is concerned with acquiring profit for the few (sometimes even to the extent that others are harmed). Thus some science is seen as supporting for-profit industry and technology that increases hothouse gases, and deliberately facilitating technology that underpins unethical practices such as the sale of high tar tobacco products in the Third World. Conversely, other science is seen as supporting such beneficial technologies as the development of largely harmless wind-turbine energy, and facilitating the development of safe technology including development of pharmaceuticals by ethically acceptable research.

One danger in the emergence of a moral conscience and the establishment of ethical positions is the danger of taking a position sometimes described as 'the high moral ground'. That is, a position of not only claiming but also believing that one knows best. If the belief that 'science' knows best in a moral sense comes together with an equally strong belief that science is the only real source of knowledge, and furthermore that it is capable of uncovering knowledge to solve most if not all of our problems, the claims being made are not only extreme but dangerous. Because, allied to the belief that science knows best – indeed, that *only* science really *knows* at all – is an almost blind faith in its capabilities and an equally almost blind rejection of alternatives (as presented in religion, law or other forms of non-scientific thought). This may be viewed as a naïve and misguided position at best or an arrogant and deceptive position at worst.

Activity 10: From science to Utopia

A view is held that science can solve all the problems of humankind. As we advance our sciences and our technologies we will eradicate disease and need, construct ideal living environments, and create a perfect and harmonious world for living.

However, such faith in science may be naïve. The term *scientism* is used to describe this. Scientism is the view that the natural sciences are the only valid sources of factual knowledge about the world (Williams 1983). There is an almost blind faith in what is viewed as hard science; science will solve all our problems and lead us into a new and better world. In our next section, we explore the limitations of such assumptions, and in the next chapter we consider how patterns of knowing other than empirical or scientific patterns may inform nursing practice.

For now, draw upon your own experience to date in clinical areas. Do you feel that there is too much faith being placed in the technologies of science? Is this more characteristic of some groups than others? In particular, compare medical and nursing staff – do they differ in their alignment to the scientific orientation, and if so why?

Science (and theory) disappointing the world

It is important to remember that particularly from the middle to latter part of the 20th century, doubts relating to science extended beyond moral concerns. Within science the movement known as positivism had exerted an influence well beyond the bounds of the laboratory and the academe. The fundamental 'positivist' position was that which saw science as a quest for real or genuine true knowledge. This could only be achieved by observing – through sensing and experiencing – how things were and how things worked in the world. In effect, the only genuine knowledge was that procured through empirical (experiential) means, by the objective identification and measurement of phenomena.

The positivist's claims for absolute truth were persuasive. They fitted well with significant scientific discoveries that greatly benefited humanity. Furthermore, the devaluing of other forms of knowledge in comparison to this persuasive position was in turn compelling. Society, having previously placed its faith in religion and law, now saw science as the route to a new Utopia. Science would eradicate poverty and disease; it would allow us to develop new technologies that would make life a veritable heaven upon earth. Consider the labour-saving devices that we have in our homes or that we carry on our person.

Unfortunately, while science led to the invention of penicillin (a life-saving antibiotic) and electricity, it also led to the invention of thalidomide (a medicine highly toxic to unborn infants) and the aforementioned nuclear armaments. Science, it was discovered, could not lead to absolute truth or the total harnessing of nature to our advantage, and indeed its products might sometimes harm us. It is not that the advantages brought by science and, its fellow traveller, technology were being discounted. These advantages were and are vitally important to the wellbeing of people and indeed all living things, and the environment within which they dwell. The impact of inventions such as antibiotics and electricity in the past is at least matched by advancing modern-day technologies such as the internet (and its application in such endeavours as distance education and telemedicine). But what is different now is the increasing realisation that the products of science and technology may be harmful and even possibly destructive on a global scale.

In the final two decades of the 20th century academics such as Anthony Giddens (1999) and Ulrich Beck (1992, 1999) wrote extensively on what was being referred to as a *risk society*. Having been concerned with (in the sense of attending to) the positive advances of science and technology, the concern increasingly turned to the risks or negative side effects of these advances. On the one hand, nuclear science produced the means of generating heat, while on the other hand it created noxious substances that would exist in increasingly large stockpiles for many centuries. Similarly, the toxic emissions from fossil fuels were increasing hothouse gases and the phenomenon of global warming. By the end of the 20th century Beck and his colleagues were already going beyond the concept of *risk society* to the idea of *global risk*. It was increasingly argued that these people-made threats involved a risk for the total planet. It is indeed only now that politicians and major Western powers are taking this seriously.

It might be suggested on the basis of the latter arguments that the relationship between science and practice is a complex one. Science, we have seen, does lead to technological advances that have a direct impact upon practice. Intercontinental air travel, modern antibiotics, high technology food processing, laser technology and automobile travel all have profound practical implications for how we live today. But the relationship is complicated and not without its negative aspects. In a sense we are deceived into the false security of a brave and bright new world. But this is an illusion. The costs of modern super-antibiotics are the ravages of superbugs and MRSA infection. The costs of increasingly available air travel are massive increases in hothouse gases and global warming. And the cost of much technology that relieves us of burdens of activity (such as physical toil) includes the negatives of sedentary living: obesity, hypertension, cardiac disease and cancers.

Activity 11: Nursing science

When we speak of the theory that may inform practice, there is an assumption that this has been derived from research. The theory we would use is *tested theory* – theory that has been shown to adequately and consistently describe, explain and predict relationships between concepts. We will return later in the book to how we test and evaluate theory.

However, while some of the knowledge that informs nursing may derive from other disciplines, much is produced within and by nursing itself. We increasingly hear people speak of nursing science.

Reflect on the concept of nursing science. Remember also our earlier issue in reflective activity 4: as nursing is a practical discipline, theoretical or propositional knowledge (so the argument ran) is of no use.

Does the term *nursing* science similarly present incompatibility? If we cannot have propositional knowledge in nursing (or at least within nursing *practice*), can we make a case for a *science* of nursing?

Finally, in your experience, has nursing science made a contribution to the actual quality of nursing practice?

Science as a positive and harnessed activity

It is important to recognise that by the latter half of the 20th century a more reasoned and realistic outlook on the limits of science had emerged. This still broadly positivistic perspective, known as *post-positivism*, adopted the more balanced view that scientific evidence can only be viewed as the *best available knowledge* until and if or when it is refuted. It will be recalled that earlier we noted Popper's work, *Conjectures and Refutations*. This perspective in a sense reinforced the link between theory (making conjectures) and practice (seeking refutations through actions based on testing those theories – i.e. research). Such outlooks are in fact definitive of the post-positivistic orientation.

Despite such reasonable positions, a forceful reaction against any form of positivism (reasonable or otherwise) emerged. Such positivism was seen as part of *modernism*, against which a *postmodernist* position arose. Postmodernism emerged in the later decades of the 20th century as essentially a reaction against the unrealistic assertions of positivism and the perceived empty promises of modernism (Lyotard 1984). The central force within postmodernism was essentially scepticism, that is, the critical questioning of the knowledge presented by science, particularly the claims (where these existed) for discovering or establishing irrefutable absolute truth. Aligned with this was the notion that knowledge is relative rather than absolute, to a greater or lesser extent context-bound or culture-specific, and often subject to multiple meanings.

In relation to its central focus – the questioning of science's absolute and exclusive claim to 'truth' – the postmodern orientation served a useful purpose. But it also carried within its orientation three fatal shortcomings:

- First, its extreme and uncompromising rejection of all constructed knowledge: according to House and Howe (1999), the postmodern critique of all knowledge in effect nullified all knowledge claims. This, some might argue, was a totally preposterous position: to be sceptical of all knowledge to the extent of rejecting it would leave us in the extreme position of believing nothing, and therefore (presumably) having no rational (knowledge) position upon which to base our actions.
- Second, by adopting an uncompromising stance in respect of *all* knowledge claims, postmodernism was in turn obliged to even question its own position. This was in fact an orientation with self-destruction built-in. By querying all knowledge claims, even its own position on 'knowledge', and offering no constructive alternative way forward, postmodernism had itself nowhere to go, no way forward. It brought the world greater scepticism, but no answers and no alternatives.

- Third, postmodernism was to an extent already tilting at imaginary windmills. It is of course the case that even today critics of science speak of its excessive positivistic shortcomings. Indeed, this is not uncommon in nursing where the tendency to lean too much upon the natural or traditional sciences is criticised and labelled positivism. However, in reality positivism as a movement had long gone by the final quarter of the 20th century, and the post-positivistic position was already taking a more balanced and reasonable position in respect of recognising the limits of science and the need to view knowledge claims in a sceptical and critical way. Indeed, it might be argued that unlike postmodernism, post-positivism contained within it a balancing critique *and* a viable way forward.

One orientation that seems to offer a way forward from what had become the dead end of postmodernism is the outlook described variously as late modernity or 'post' modernity (although this latter term runs the risk of being confused with postmodernism). Terms such as neo-modernity and reflexive modernity have also been used. This orientation, while subject to the same lack of consensus and disputations as many other such terms, involved the extension of a post-positivistic viewpoint that was essentially a more balanced view of the advances of society, particularly within science and technology. This is characterised by the following claims or often-identified late modernity positions:

- *Balance*: balanced and critical outlook on the limits of science.
- *Openness*: recognition of the validity of other forms of knowing, and a rejection of the dominance of specific knowledge forms that rest exclusively on specific empirical orientations. Also, an openness to questioning scientific knowledge and accepting the importance of refutation as a means of strengthening rather than attacking scientific knowledge.
- *Ethical deportment*: an increasing moral consciousness that acknowledges the ethical responsibility of science as extending beyond narrow conceptions of research ethics (often limited to concerns about the truthfulness of science claims). There is recognition of the responsibility to translate science into beneficial outcomes, and an acceptance of the responsibility to proactively identify, publicly expose and rigorously combat the harmful outcomes of science. Here, we return to the idea of a risk society that we considered earlier. This is the recognition that science has indeed produced great benefits for mankind, but a growing realisation that it has also created great risks. The spread of noxious substances ranging from insecticides to tobacco and the growing threat from global warming are just two instances we have already referred to. The threats of

burgeoning globalism identified by Giddens (1999) and the global risks cited by Beck (1999) as discussed earlier bear witness to this situation. The ethical orientation increasingly emerging within science is a global ethic that extends to a more proactive involvement in containing risk.

- *Reflexivity*: a growing recognition that what is knowable is less static and more subject to constant change than may previously have been the case. This in fact requires a movement from a position of *reflection* on what is (or was in the past) knowable, to a more *reflexive* orientation to dynamic changing processes. As the argument runs here, such is the dynamic and changing nature of the world that our past knowledge and previous experiences are of limited value in addressing new and previously unencountered phenomena and the problems they present. We must therefore develop reflexive approaches, wherein the nature of what we encounter challenges us to respond appropriately.

Conclusion

We have concerned ourselves in this chapter with how practice and theory are related. A fundamental and underlying question is (by definition binary in nature): Does our practice derive from theory? And does our theory derive from our practice?

The questions are not simple. We can return to our opening quotation from Thomas Merton (1969) again. Once we start to explore the issues, we become aware of inconsistencies and lack of clarity.

If we define theory in terms of it being an aspect of science, we are thrust into the relationship between science and practice. Then, we realise that science also incorporates within its meaning an empirical dimension (recall that we spoke of theory as the thinking/postulating part of science, and research as the doing/testing part). We are thus thrust into the related relationship between research and practice. Suddenly we are faced with a quest that initially seemed contained (the relationship between theory and practice) but now raises questions in respect of:

- the theory–practice relationship
- the science–practice relationship
- the research–practice relationship.

Now, if we pause here for a moment, we will realise that the above relationships commence with the premise that theory is accepted as an element of science. However, what if that is rejected? What if theory is seen as unscientific conjecture? We are now faced with a new set of concerns, which really need to be addressed before considering the aforementioned three relationships. These are:

- the theory–science relationship
- the theory–research relationship
- the idea of theory not being a scientific construct at all.

Perhaps, when we have sorted out these six concerns, we can then attempt to clarify the theory–practice issue. But wait a moment. What of practice? What do we understand by this? Now we have a further set of concerns, only some of which include:

- practice as practical as opposed to theoretical
- practical as real world, theory as divorced from real world
- practice as doing
- practical knowledge as atheoretical know-how.

We now have up to ten concerns that frame our original apparently simple-enough question. And without a doubt we could add some more! We will now recognise the importance of Merton's (1969) statement in the opening quotation to this chapter. We *do* always need to return to our earlier assumptions, to again review our definitions. However, we might be forgiven for suggesting that if we proceed to do this we make ourselves even more confused, we end up going around in circles, and we answer none of our questions.

It is important not to get despondent here. If this chapter has done little more than demonstrate that the simple questions raised are complex and multifaceted, and if it has made you more sceptical and critical about superficial statements on the relationship between theory and practice, it has achieved a lot and, in reality, so have you. Furthermore, later in the book, and particularly in Chapter 6, we take up this issue again (for example, we extend the argument by considering the relationship between research, theory and practice).

Fortunately, we can add some comments about the relationship between theory and practice. These may seem limited and unimpressive. However, assuming you have worked your way through the chapter, they were positions hard come by. We can present them as such:

1   In one sense, practice is characterised by atheoretical knowledge that we have termed know-how.
2   The relationship between such know-how and theory is mainly to do with understanding the nature of know-how. Once we recognise its nature, its true sophistication and its importance to nursing

we will nurture and respect this know-how, particularly as it exists at levels of expertise.

3 Theoretical or propositional knowledge is equally important in practice, as the means by which we describe, explain and predict situations in the practice setting, and prescribe or make choices on the basis of this knowledge.

4 Importantly, we must recognise the close complementary relationship between theory and practice, including the knowledge of practical doing that we term *know-how*. We must know *what* is the best thing to do in practice situations (through knowledge derived from tested theory) and we must know *how* to do it (through the development of practical know-how).

5 We recognise different levels of theory in terms of abstraction – from specific micro theory that is largely testable hypotheses, and middle range theory that is specific enough from which to formulate such hypotheses, to the most abstract forms of grand theory that map out or frame the knowledge field (in our case, nursing).

6 There are different sources of theoretical knowledge and it can be seen as: emerging from other disciplines through being adopted or adapted to the nursing purpose, or emerging from the nursing field itself as theory derived from practice, or indeed from all these sources (e.g. where the practice context helps us adapt non-nursing theory to the nursing context).

7 Knowledge used in practice must be thoroughly tested and presented as the best information or evidence available, as in evidence-based practice. Theory, even where it is constructed from such reliable evidence, must also be tested for its fitness for purpose.

8 Not all knowledge of a rational or propositional nature fits in with the view of theory as science, and there is a need to recognise that other knowledge forms (sometimes also defined as theory in a wider meaning of the term) – e.g. ethical or aesthetic forms of knowledge – must also inform our practice.

9 We recognise the distinction between theory and theorising, and also the case for recognising that we all theorise (attempt to make sense of our environment) as a fundamental characteristic of being human.

10 Given that nurses themselves theorise about their practice, we recognise that there is no such thing as practice *without* theory. We therefore recognise the need to ensure that this valuable, context-bound theory is also nurtured, and where possible explicated and tested.

11 Insofar as nurses themselves theorise, and are also presented with theory that may inform their practice, there is a need to develop

within nursing practice a sceptical and critical approach to theory, particularly where it has not or can not be adequately tested.

12 We have demonstrated that theory is derived from science and in turn contributes to science. To the extent that theory is indeed sometimes recognised as part of science (the conjectural, creative part, that relates to and indeed guides the doing or research part), there is a need to view critically what has and can be achieved by science and theory.

13 There is the particular need to recognise the risks that have emerged from science, some of a global nature, and the ways in which these risks impact upon our practice.

14 This need to look to the future that is unfurling and how we might respond indicates the importance of embracing grand theory perspectives that were perhaps rejected previously, for it is these that are designed to look towards our horizons and the new ways forward.

Activity 12: Final words, final reflections

This is an extensive and indeed extremely dense chapter. It is one of the longest in the book. It addresses perhaps one of the most fundamental of all nursing questions: the relationship between theory and practice.

Your journey through the chapter and its reflective activities of course extended your reading and thinking considerably. It may be on the basis of this that you feel you would modify some of the above summary statements, or that you might even add to them.

Given the nature of the chapter, it might be useful now or at some subsequent stage to re-read the chapter and your own notes from the various exercises. After that, review the above 14 points, extending and/or refining them as you see fit.

Summary

The relationship between theory and practice was explored in detail. It was argued that while some aspects of practice derive from practical know-how rather than propositional knowledge, other aspects depend upon sound theory derived from the best rational thinking and empirical evidence. The definitional statements of theory were extended into classifying theory in terms of increasing complexity (as in descriptive, explanatory, predictive and prescriptive theory), and increasingly abstract properties (as in grand theory, middle range theory and hypotheses). The relationship was further explored in terms of how theory may inform practice and how in turn practice may inform theory and contribute to theory construction. This discussion was carried forward into the issue of the relationship between science and practice, given that theory is most often recognised as a part of science. The chapter ends with summary statements that characterise these relationships, and the student reader is invited to elaborate upon these.

Knowing and Knowledge: Importance for Nursing

'If you dissemble sometimes your knowledge of that you thought you know, you shall be thought, another time, to know that you know not.'

Francis Bacon (1561–1626)

Outline of content

Knowledge and knowing are defined, by introducing defining terms and proceeding to consider how knowledge is constructed. Rationalism, empiricism and critical thinking are presented as means of producing knowledge. The influences of positivism, logical-positivism, post-positivism, critical theory and constructivism on how we perceive and construct knowledge are explored. Different categories of knowledge and different patterns of knowing in nursing are presented. The roles of research and reasoning in constructing nursing knowledge are outlined.

The quotation from Bacon shows that we should always challenge what we know and take little for granted. However, there are distinct differences between knowing and knowledge. A useful starting point for this chapter would be to define these terms. According to Chinn and Kramer (2004) *knowing* refers to the individual human processes of experiencing and comprehending the self and the world in ways that can be brought to some level of conscious awareness. This implies that because it alters with experience, knowing is always in a state of flux.

Notice that it is also about how we comprehend ourselves and the world in which we live. Therefore, as we mature and as the work changes, our knowing also changes. A more esoteric view of knowing comes from the Jewish *Talmud*:

> 'the child in the womb of his mother looks from one end of the world to the other and knows all the teaching, but the instant he comes in contact with the air of earth an angel strikes him on the mouth and he forgets everything'. (cited in Levine 1994)

But not all is forgotten; we all have instincts such as blinking, sucking and eye dilatation. These ways of surviving are underpinned by instinctive knowing.

Chinn and Kramer (2004) defined *knowledge* as simply the knowing that we can share with or communicate to others. This implies that there may be knowledge that we will not share or cannot communicate to others and so this, by their definition, is not knowledge! However, if you share or communicate your knowing with others this 'knowledge' becomes part of their store of knowing. Similarly, if they share knowledge with us it becomes part of our store of knowing. In nursing we share knowledge in many different ways such as through speaking, use of the written word and through our behaviour. We obtain knowledge through our five senses: hearing, seeing, touching, smelling and tasting. There is also a view supported by Martha Rogers (1980), the American nurse theorist, that we have a sixth sense which enables us to practise competently. We have already referred to this 'tacit knowing' in Chapter 2 but it deserves to be explored in more detail later in this chapter.

Philosophies of knowledge

In the main there are many philosophical views on how knowledge develops; nonetheless, three will be explained here: rationalism, empiricism and historicism.

Rationalism

Rationalism has its stem in *ratio*, the Latin word for 'reason'. Charles Darwin stated that of all the faculties of the human mind, reason stands at the summit (Barnhart & Barnhart 1976). It is a philosophy of science which emphasises the role that reason has to play in the development of knowledge and the discovery of truth. Its philosophical roots are of interest.

Rationalism is founded on the idea that theorists, without access to data obtained through the senses, can generate theory through mental reasoning. They do this by formulating propositions through theorising how one concept could be related to others. This 'armchair theorising' has been ridiculed, mainly because of the absence of hard data. Nonetheless, the absence of data has not stopped people taking such theories seriously. For example, Freud used rationalism to develop his theories of psychoanalysis; he had very little data to support his theories on the Oedipus complex, or the id, ego and superego (Freud 1949).

In essence, rationalists theorise without data and then experiments are set up in the real world to see if the theory can be collaborated. This is best described as the 'theory then research' approach (Reynolds 1971) and can also be called deductive or *a priori* reasoning. Einstein's theory of relativity was formed many years before methods were available to test it, so this is perhaps the best-known example of the development of such knowledge.

Rationalism as an approach to knowledge development can be traced to Rene Descartes (1596–1650), the 17th-century French philosopher and mathematician introduced to you in Chapter 2. He spent most of his adult life in Holland and influenced other famous rationalists such as Antoine Arnauld (1612–94), Benedict de Spinoza (1632–77) and Gottfried von Leibniz (1646–1716).

Nine years before his death Descartes published a book entitled *Meditations on First Philosophy* (1641). This was to influence the development of knowledge for the next 300 years. Perhaps the best word to signify his contribution to rationalism is 'doubt'. He realised that to arrive at new knowledge you must put former opinions and experiences in doubt. When we do this we can build knowledge from first principles (Stokes 2004).

As noted above, most of our knowledge comes from our senses. However, Descartes noted that the senses can play tricks on us. For example, we may think something looks cold but when we touch it, it is hot, or we may believe that a creaking floorboard or a branch blowing against a window is an intruder. Descartes considered sensory deceptions such as these and reflected that they could be the work of a malignant being, a demon whose role is to fool us by sending us false sensory information. Such misconceptions are often used to good effect in Hollywood films such as *The Matrix* (Wachowski & Wachowski 1999).

When Descartes reasoned that all his knowledge may be false through being fooled by the demon, he came to doubt all that he previously held to be true and to exist. He even began to doubt his own existence. However, he realised that there was one thing that the demon could not falsify. He reasoned that when he thinks, he must exist or else he would not be able to think. Such reasoning led him to the one certain piece of true knowledge referred to in Chapter 2, 'Cogito, ergo sum', (I think, therefore I am). Following this, he held that by means of reason alone, knowledge and certain universal self-evident truths could be discovered, from which the sciences could then be deductively derived.

Descartes was a devout Catholic and he reasoned that God created two classes of substance that make up the whole of reality. One class was thinking substances, or minds, and the other was extended substances, or bodies. This mind–matter split, or Cartesian dualism, is based on the assumption that we are rational individuals with rational minds and that our minds are divorced from our bodies and from other matter.

Rationalism as a philosophy of science was very influential. Descartes' mind–body split underpins much of the medical model. Physicians were often trained to look for anatomical signs and physiological symptoms and come up with a diagnosis. The fact that the patient worked in a highly stressed job or that he was worried about having cancer were not given the slightest consideration. Similarly, when nurses assess patients objectively from a physical and pathological perspective while ignoring their thoughts, emotions and feelings they are practising Cartesian dualism. We still hear experienced nurses referring to a 'coronary' or a 'stroke' being admitted!

We have alluded to the work of Karl Popper (1902–94) earlier. He was one of a group of philosophers known as the New Scientists and was influenced by Descartes. As we stated, Popper argued that the way to true knowledge was by conjecture (developing theory through reason) and refutation (testing the theory through rigorous research to see if it could be proved false). To him, the mark of a scientific theory was whether it made predictions that could be proved false through testing (Popper 1965).

Empiricism

In contrast to rationalists, empiricists believe that knowledge is derived entirely from sensory experience. In other words if something cannot be perceived through the five senses, it does not exist. As distinct from rationalism, empiricism denies the possibility of spontaneous ideas or *a priori* reasoning as a predecessor to scientific knowledge. Rather, empiricists formulate concepts and propositions that attempt to explain the phenomena they have experienced. These propositions may be turned into hypotheses which can be tested through experimental research. The end result is knowledge in the form of theory. Empiricism can be described as the 'research then theory' approach (Reynolds 1971) and because the theory comes last, this type of knowledge development can also be called inductive or *a posteriori* reasoning.

The origin of empiricism can be traced to a number of English philosophers including John Locke (1632–1704) and David Hume (1711–76). Locke was the first to put forward empiricist principles in his *Essay Concerning Human Understanding*. He spent 20 years writing this book postulating on how the mind collects, organises and makes judgements based on all the data that come to us through our senses. He had read Descartes but had rejected the rationalist philosophy as not helping to explain human understanding. For Locke there can be no innate knowledge: rather everything we know must be gained from experience. To him, knowledge was derived from the outside world writing on our minds through our senses. Therefore, he envisioned the mind at birth to be a blank slate, what he referred to as *tabula rasa* (Stokes 2004). As the child develops, this slate is written on by experience.

Locke distinguished between primary and secondary qualities. Primary qualities are objective and include shape, solidity, number and motion. In contrast, secondary qualities are more subjective and include colour, smell and taste. The reason why they are termed secondary is that they are produced in our minds by the effect of primary qualities on our senses. To him, primary qualities really exist in the world and secondary qualities exist in our minds. For example, the primary qualities of a cancer can be observed and its size, shape and position measured. Less important for empiricists would be the pain, fear and distress that the cancer causes for the patient. These would be labelled secondary qualities by Locke. Put very simplistically, from an empiricist perspective cancer biologists would mainly be concerned with the size, position and type of cancerous growth, whereas nurses would mainly be concerned with the effect the growth was having on the patient and his family. Neither may be right but the philosophies underpinning the education and training of different health professionals may go some way to explain these different perspectives.

Ninety-four years after Locke's death, the French philosopher Auguste Comte (1798–1857), gave empiricism a new twist. He is best remembered for being a student activist and an anti-establishment figure and he saw science as a means of changing and possibly overthrowing political movements. One of his many legacies is that he founded the discipline of sociology as a means of applying the methods of science to the study of people and society.

In his six-volume work *Course of Positive Philosophy* (1830–42), Comte used the term 'positive' philosophy to differentiate it from the negative philosophy which he believed underpinned woolly and metaphysical thinking. Adopting such a 'positivist' approach meant that through the use of robust scientific methods human problems would be solved and social conditions improved. In his view, scientists should focus on ordering confirmable observations in a rigorous manner; this alone should constitute human knowledge.

Activity 1: Exploring knowledge

In this chapter we carry forward in more detail issues about knowledge first encountered back in Chapter 1 and to an extent also in Chapter 2. Now, we recognise that knowledge is shared and accepted knowledge is derived from different sources – mainly rational thinking (reasoning) and experience (formally encountered in empirical methods).

Reflect a little further on these issues by exploring the literature. Seek definitions of: knowledge, rationalism and empiricism. Consider how rationalism and empiricism are encountered in nursing practice.

Comte also identified a hierarchy of six sciences that had been founded on systematic observation (astronomy, biology, chemistry, mathematics, physics and sociology). These formed the 'gold standard' against which other disciplines would be judged. In contrast, he perceived subjective approaches to knowledge development as not being meaningful pursuits, and so reflection and intuition as a basis for gaining knowledge were shunned and denigrated by the positivists.

Throughout his life Comte was plagued by mental health problems and on occasions he attempted suicide. In his later years his mental illness returned and with it a softening of his views regarding positivism. For instance, in some of his last writings, such as *The Catechism of Positive Religion*, he stated that the intellect should be the servant of the heart!

Nonetheless, it is for his earlier work on positivism that Comte will be best remembered. Many scientists argued that it was the only true source of knowledge. In essence, the doctrine involved the following logic: our minds interpret the world through our senses, and because the world is subject to the laws of science, events outside the mind can be observed, described, explained and predicted. Therefore, to make sense of the outside world all we have to do is to observe it and undertake experiments to test hypotheses formulated from such observations. For positivists, objective truth exists and the goal of science is to go out and discover it; in their view this forms our knowledge base.

At the turn of the 20th century a group of philosophers formed an organisation called 'the Vienna Circle', which included Moritz Schlick (1882–1936) and Ludwig Wittgenstein (1889–1951). They built on Comte's ideas and coined the term 'logical positivism', placing an even stronger emphasis on the importance of induction and scientific verification (Emden 1991).

For most of the first half of the 20th century 'respected' scientists adopted the logical positivist view of science. However, the philosophical force behind logical positivism dissipated just before World War Two when most of its supporters left Nazi Germany and Austria. Today, in the first decade of the 21st century it is seen as a spent force in scientific enquiry.

Nursing did not escape being touched by positivism and Suppe and Jacox (1985) asserted that it had a strong influence on the development of nursing theory. However, Afaf Meleis (1985, 1991, 1997, 2007) did not uncover much evidence of this and Ann Whall (1989) found even less when she studied nursing practice guides for the years 1950–70. Nonetheless, as alluded to in Chapter 2, the reductionism, classification and categorical ordering that are hallmarks of positivism can be seen in how several nurse theorists reduce individuals to a number of activities of living, adaptation modes or self-care capabilities.

Popper (1965), initially a supporter of the Vienna Circle, began to reject induction as a scientific approach and replaced their emphasis on verification with his principle of falsification. In other words, theories should not be tested to see if they can be supported, rather, they should be tested to see if they can be proved false. If you test a theory 19 times and it holds true it may not hold true on the 20th occasion. To Popper, we can learn much more from the 20th test than from the previous 19. An example would be if you were to construct a kite and test it to see if it will fly. It may fly perfectly the first 20 times you try it but on the next few attempts it crash lands! To Popper this lack of reliability would be an important discovery and you would have to go back to the drawing board to redesign the kite.

Later in his life he began to question the logical positivists' desire to reject subjectivity as a way of knowing. In what could be seen as a 'road to Damascus' change, Popper admitted that there was a place for intuition and imagination when one is using scientific empiricism!

Today, thanks to philosophers like Popper, logical positivism has been replaced by post-positivist empiricism, a much milder form of positivism. Gortner (1993) supported the use of this form of empiricism in the development of nursing science. She felt it was unfortunate that it was still being tarnished in the literature by being confused with logical positivism. Modern empiricists accept the shortcomings of verification and recognise that the world is complex and some behaviours and events can be reduced for study purposes and some cannot.

Empiricism is still highly regarded as a scientific approach in the physical sciences of biology, physics and chemistry. All of the many experiments, quasi-experiments and randomised controlled trials carried out within nursing are clearly based upon empiricism. In 1993, when referring to nursing theories, Gortner argued that Roy's (1989) theory 'reflects clearly the thinking of an empiricist scholar' (Gortner 1993: 481). The same can be said of the theories of Orem (1980, 1985, 1995), Neuman (1995) and Henderson (1966).

Historicism

So far we have dealt with knowledge that is objective and can be perceived through the senses. Much of this knowledge can be measured. You will recall our story in Chapter 1 of the Italian astronomer Galileo Galilei (1564–1642). He maintained that we should 'measure what is measurable, count what is countable and what is not countable, make countable'. However, there are many phenomena of interest to nurses that cannot be measured. How would you calibrate compassion, measure empathy, or quantify a presence? True rationalist or empirical principles could not be applied to these. The philosophy of science best suited to this perspective is called historicism.

Historicism recognises that we are all influenced by our different histories and different experiences, values and beliefs. From these influences we construct our own realities and we interpret events from this construction. Therefore, another term for this view of science is the interpretative-constructionist approach.

Consider the following example: two nurses can observe an elderly patient getting out of bed and interpret it differently. One may believe that the patient is dependent and in danger of falling and should not attempt to get out of bed. The other may perceive the patient to be gaining independence and therefore is pleased that they are getting out of bed.

These nurses observe the same clinical phenomenon, yet past experience, reflection and intuition lead them to understand and interpret it differently. Furthermore, each may have a personal or internationally accepted theory which structures what they perceive. Such 'theoretical baggage' influences how we attempt to understand what we experience. So, to different people, reality (and knowledge of that reality) is often a personal thing, the product of individual reflection, perception, perspective and purpose rather than being static and objective.

Realising this, philosophers such as Kuhn (1977), Toulmin (1972) and Feyerabend (1977) challenged the positivist view and stressed the importance of history and perception in the development of science. They rejected the idea of there being objective truths, arguing instead that the development of knowledge is a dynamic process and so there are no final and permanent truths.

How science develops

Prior to Thomas Kuhn's book *The Structure of Scientific Revolutions* (1977) many scientists, particularly from the empiricist/positivist traditions, believed that different research studies built upon one another in a progression of the science leading eventually to ultimate truth. In contrast, Kuhn (1922–96) asserted that science progressed through a series of *revolutionary* steps. After each revolution there is a period of 'normal science' where a particular paradigm (remember we called this a worldview in Chapter 1) reigns supreme and scholars accept it as a basis for knowledge and truth. Rejecting this paradigm during a period of normal science would be frowned upon by the scientific community. However, according to Kuhn this paradigm is eventually questioned. This may be because it fails to deal adequately with some new phenomenon, or a new, more powerful paradigm has greater explanatory power. As more evidence accumulates to show that the old way of thinking has outlived its usefulness a 'paradigm shift' occurs. Kuhn maintained that paradigm shifts are not cumulative and the new paradigm is not built on the previous paradigm. The new paradigm becomes the focus for a new period of normal science (Stokes 2004).

One example of this would be Ptolemy's teaching that the Sun orbited the Earth. This paradigm held sway for centuries in what Kuhn would call 'normal science'. However, when Copernicus (1473–1543) challenged this with his theory that the Earth moved around the Sun, a paradigm shift took place. Other examples include Newton's theory of gravity being replaced by Einstein's theory of relativity, or the contemporary focus on community care as opposed to institutional care for those with mental health problems. Paradigm shifts occurred because the old paradigms were not able to explain new experiences or solve new problems. The views of Kuhn did much to undermine the empirical/positivist view of science.

Larry Laudan (1977) challenged Kuhn's view that knowledge development was a revolutionary process. Rather, he believed that knowledge was developed in an evolutionary way with new knowing being influenced by previous knowing. This *evolutionary* approach of Laudan is an attractive one for nurses because it recognised a pluralistic view to knowledge development and application. After all, the problems facing nursing are forever changing and staff must select the theory and paradigm that is best suited to solving these problems.

More recently, Afaf Meleis (1985), the US-based Egyptian nurse metatheorist, argued that the revolutionary and evolutionary approaches to knowledge development are too simplistic on their own to explain nursing's experience of knowledge development. She coined the term 'convolution' to explain how nursing knowledge has developed. She maintained that nursing as a discipline has progressed not through evolution or revolution but through a *convolutionary* series of peaks, troughs, detours and backward steps and a series of crises. This gives the impression that knowledge development in nursing is confusing and uncoordinated. There may be some truth in this as nursing is still a young scientific discipline, one which Kuhn (1977) may place in a pre-paradigmatic stage of development.

The move to phenomenology

Edmund Husserl (1859–1938) was a German philosopher and the founder of phenomenology. Phenomenology is the study of the meaning of phenomena to a particular individual and a way of understanding people from the way things appear to them (George 2001). In contrast to the empiricists and positivists, Husserl believed that science involved the exploration of perceptions, judgements, beliefs and other mental processes. He argued that, because of its refusal to count anything other than observable entities and objective reality, positivism was not capable of dealing with human experience. He maintained that one way to truth was to consider the essence of things, and the best way of noting this was to explore what meaning the mind has for that thing (Husserl 1962).

The task of 'phenomenology' is to discover what life experiences are like for people. Understanding their 'lived experience' requires the use of reflection, which is the basis of phenomenology. While Descartes was sceptical about the external world (see above), Husserl was sceptical about self-knowledge. Therefore, he recommended that phenomenologists should 'bracket existence'. This meant that when they are exploring the essence of an occurrence or an event they should suspend previous views and influences as this would merely distort their true perception of it.

Martin Heidegger (1889–1976), a student of Husserl, maintained that as a way of generating knowledge, phenomenology should make manifest what is hidden in everyday taken-for-granted experience. He disagreed with Husserl's idea that an observer can 'bracket existence'. Rather he argued that prior experiences and influences may be used positively in a phenomenological study.

Hermeneutics, a branch of phenomenology much influenced by Heidegger, is based upon the idea that all texts and human activities are filled with meaning and can be subject to rigorous interpretations. Therefore, within hermeneutics, to know is to understand through interpretation. In Heidegger's philosophical view the understanding of phenomena is not about measuring, analysing and classifying. Once more the hard science is being softened to take account of meaning and perception rather than detached quantification (Stokes 2004). Here softening is not about being less rigorous or systematic.

Activity 2: Sourcing knowledge

Thus far, we have noted that knowledge may come from rational thinking or empirical inquiry. The latter may involve a quantitative observing and measuring of the world or things in it, or a more qualitative form of enquiry that seeks meaning rather than measures.

Briefly review each of these sources of knowledge. Consider whether any or all are needed in nursing, and if so why. Give one example of how each may be used in practice. The three forms are: rational thinking, empirical quantitative inquiry, and phenomenological or hermeneutic inquiry.

Critical science

We referred above to the Vienna Circle which was a group that believed staunchly in logical positivism. Contemporaneously, a rival group existed called the Frankfurt School. It was located in the University of Frankfurt am Main in Germany and was established by Max Horkheimer who became its director in 1930. The Frankfurt School gathered together dissident Marxists and was very much anti-positivist in its teachings. They saw positivism as an inappropriate way of viewing knowledge development in the social sciences; they favoured the critical science approach.

Critical science is also a variant of phenomenology but goes further; stressing that meanings should not be merely elicited but should be open to criticism (Habermas 1971). It is a very political philosophy and an attractive approach for those nurses who wish to leave behind subservience to the male-dominated health service. It has given rise to feminist research methodologies and action research and as such may be perceived as a science of freedom. There are three major concepts within critical theory (Emden 1991):

- *Enlightenment*: knowledge of self in relation to the world and education of the oppressed in terms of their potential capacity to bring about change;
- *Empowerment*: social transformation through some form of educative process;
- *Emancipation*: a state of reflective clarity where people have a sense of themselves and can determine freely and collectively the directions they should take in life.

Critical theory's focus on education, enlightenment, emancipation, empowerment, critique and change is an attractive perspective to many nurses and is supported by the increase in the number of feminist and action research studies in nursing in recent years.

How do nurses know?

Most nurses have long accepted that people undergoing care deserve interventions which are based on sound knowledge. In the mid 19th century, Florence Nightingale (1859) argued that nurses required a body of knowledge that was distinct from that of physicians. Because of her educational background she was aware of the positivist view of science and was a proponent of that philosophy. She excelled in statistical analysis of data and the research approaches she used in studying conditions in the British army tended to favour a positivist methodology. In fact, she was more famous for this in the mid 19th century than she was for her influence on nursing.

Nightingale was probably the first nurse theorist. Fifty years after her death, other nurse theorists became committed to the same principle of developing an organised body of nursing knowledge for the purpose of guiding practice. One such theorist, Dorothy Johnson (1968), asserted that 'no profession can long exist without making explicit its theoretical basis for practice so that this knowledge can be communicated, tested and expanded' (p. 291). She further argued that society will only give nurses the authority and responsibility for practice if there is proof that they possess the knowledge required to do the job. Readers will recognise the link with the current evidence-based practice movement.

Johnson (1968) asserted that knowledge does not belong to any one group or discipline. She maintained that just because one discipline discovers or creates knowledge does not confer the right of ownership. Therefore, a body of knowledge formulated within a specific discipline belongs to the world at large and as a result there is no nursing knowledge, merely knowledge that nurses use in a particular way.

Know-how, know-that and know-why knowledge

Schön (1987) described the 'high hard ground' world of academia and the 'swampy lowlands' of practice. Knowledge in the former is more theoretic and abstract while knowledge in the latter is continually altering in complexity, instability and uncertainty. Knowledge in the 'swamp' is also full of value conflicts (Meave 1994).

We introduced you to the two types of knowledge described by Rhyl (1963) as 'know-how knowledge' and 'know-that knowledge'. You will recall that the former is skills based and involves knowing the mechanics of how to do something. This may include how to use the internet or how to drive a car. But you may know how to do these tasks without knowing how a computer is programmed or the mechanical theory of the internal combustion engine. In nursing, much of 'know-how knowledge' is perceived as our 'art' and therefore has its roots in historicism. In contrast, 'know-that knowledge' has its basis in theory and empirical research and is often perceived as our 'science'.

The value system underlying 'know-that knowledge' is aligned to the philosophy of empiricism and is often held in much higher regard than know-how knowledge. However, a rift exists between the know-how knowledge of clinical practice and the know-that knowledge taught in the classroom (Chambers 1995). Practitioners are continually being urged to implement research findings with the hidden assumption that what they are doing in practice (know-how knowledge) is incorrect and perhaps even wasteful and detrimental to clients.

Many nurses think that nursing students are too theoretical and are not fit to practise (UKCC 1999). There is a perception that nursing students know the theory of why they should undertake care processes (strong know-that knowledge), but they have difficulty doing so (weak know-how knowledge). Conversely, there is a perception that many practising nurses excel intuitively in undertaking care processes (strong know-how knowledge) while they often have difficulty in explaining how they know how to do certain tasks (weak know-that knowledge).

This is a perennial paradox in nursing and has been at the root of many reorganisations of nursing education worldwide.

This may be explained partly by the findings of Patricia Benner (1983). She conducted a well-cited study using a phenomenological approach. She found that novices in nursing needed quite rigid rules, procedures and guidelines to enable them to feel secure within clinical situations. Expert nurses, on the other hand, often found such rules an unnecessary encumbrance and mostly practised intuitively. It is particularly interesting that in many instances these expert nurses were unable to precisely explain why or how they knew certain things.

As alluded to previously, Polanyi (1958) identified this phenomenon and called it 'tacit knowing' to distinguish it from 'explicit knowing'. Slevin (1995) defined tacit knowledge as a high degree of capacity to function with expertise without having to think, explain or problem solve, indeed often being unable to explain why it is 'just known' that something is right in a particular situation. This definition places tacit knowing firmly within the category of know-how knowledge.

Perhaps if theory was based upon know-how knowledge it might be easier for practitioners to accept it as being appropriate for their practice. One way of achieving this is to use a phenomenological approach to knowledge development. From above you recall that phenomenology encourages the generation of theoretical knowledge through exploring the meaning and experience of, among other things, 'know-how' practice. This can lead to the generation of new theories having their foundations in the 'know-how' knowledge of practice. Practitioners could also bridge the theory–practice gap by being encouraged and supported to apply research and theory to their practice. In this way know-how knowledge would be the conduit for putting 'know-that' knowledge into practice.

However, there is another dimension that is seldom explored and that is know-why knowledge. This goes a stage further than know-how and know-that knowledge. For example, a nurse may Know How to position a patient who has chronic obstructive airways disease so that they are more comfortable. The nurse may also Know That the research indicates that this is the best way to nurse patients with this disease. But there is another dimension to this scenario; the nurse may Know Why this is the case. They know that if such patients are nursed flat, their abdominal organs will press on their diaphragm and this will increase pressure on their lungs and cause greater difficulty with breathing. It would seem that when providing care many nurses have know-how knowledge, fewer have know-that knowledge and fewer still have know-why knowledge.

You will note that know-why knowledge is closely related to Dickoff and James's (1968) higher levels of theory as discussed in Chapter 2.

Categories of knowing

Pierce (1957) identified seven ways of knowing. These were:

- knowing through being told by an authority figure
- knowing through unverified hearsay
- knowing through the experience of trial and error
- knowing indirectly through past experiences (history)
- knowing by unverified belief
- knowing through spiritual or divine understanding
- knowing through intuition.

This covers the historicism and rationalism philosophies of knowing, but not empiricism.

More recently, Kerlinger (1986) addressed this. He asserted that the way to truth is through rigorous research, involving the identification of variables within hypotheses and subjecting them to experimental manipulation. Here 'hard evidence' is required in order to be certain that something is or is not true. You will note that this reflects a positivist viewpoint. But Kerlinger also identified what he thought were less respectable ways of knowing. These are tenacity, authority and *a priori*.

Knowing through *tenacity* is knowing something because it has always been believed to be true. Knowing though *authority* is knowing something because a respected or authoritative person said so. Knowing through *a priori* is knowing something because reason tells you it is true. The end result of each of these ways of knowing is knowledge; what differs is how the knowledge is acquired.

To illustrate Kerlinger's approach we could take the example of the knowledge that providing information to patients preoperatively will ensure better postoperative recovery. Nurses may believe this to be true because 'it has always been done this way' (tenacity) or the ward sister told them so (authority) or that it is reasonable to assume that if a person gets information they will be less anxious (*a priori*). You could also have identified Kerlinger's preferred positivist way of obtaining knowledge; nurses provide patients with information preoperatively because this practice was proven through the collection of empirical data or through studying the results of well-validated empirical research into preoperative preparation (see Boore 1978).

Like all physical scientists, authors like Pierce and Kerlinger feel comfortable building hierarchies of knowledge. In Kerlinger's scheme the scientific empiricist method is supreme and intuitive knowledge occupies a lowly position. For a practice discipline like nursing this is an inappropriate way of viewing the development of knowledge. Such hierarchies are seen in textbooks on evidence-based practice. For example, in 1997 Muir Gray identified what he called the hierarchy of evidence (Table 3.1) (Muir Gray 1997).

You will notice that the top four levels are really about counting and that this predilection has its roots in empiricism.

It is not unusual to hear the mantra that randomised controlled trials are the gold standard, the most highly prized source of knowledge. This is a false assumption as it depends on what knowledge you are pursuing. If we wanted to know the possible causes of diabetes, then the randomised controlled trial may well be the gold standard. However, if we wanted to know the effect of diabetes on patients and their families, then the gold standard may be a phenomenological study.

According to this hierarchy, word of mouth is not regarded as good evidence. This is not the case in all professions. In the legal profession such evidence is highly valued and word of mouth is sufficient to put a person in jail for a long time, or in some countries be executed. In contrast, such sources are denigrated in most textbooks and articles about evidence in nursing. Perhaps it might be more useful for a new hierarchy (Table 3.2) to be proposed.

As with the previous hierarchy, this one also has inherent problems. How can you decide whether a patient's preference comes above or below the experience of nurses? It depends on circumstances; hierarchies belong to the world of positivist quantification and the quality of knowledge required to care should not be tied to the quality of a research design.

Table 3.1 The hierarchy of evidence (Muir Gray 1997).

Level I	Meta-analysis of a series of randomised controlled trials
Level II	At least one well-designed randomised controlled trial
Level III	At least one controlled study without randomisation
Level IV	Well-designed non-experimental studies
Level V	Case reports, clinical examples, opinions of experts

Table 3.2 The new hierarchy of evidence.

Level I	Opinion and views of experts
Level II	Patients' preferences and narrative accounts
Level III	Nurses' experiences
Level IV	Results of qualitative studies and quality improvement/audit activities
Level V	Results of quantitative research

Carper's ways of knowing in nursing

In 1978 in the first article in the first issue of a new US journal, *Advances in Nursing Science*, Barbara Carper identified four patterns of knowing in nursing. It proved to be a seminal paper and the four patterns of knowing were: *empirics*, the science of nursing; *aesthetics*, the art of nursing; *ethics*, moral knowing; and *personal knowing*.

Empirics

By now you can probably predict the type of knowing that 'empirics' would signify. According to Carper 'empirics' represents the knowing that is obtained by rigorous observation or measurement. It provides knowledge that is *verifiable, objective, factual* and *research based*. This is the type of quantifiable and objective evidence seen in levels 1 to 4 of Muir Grey's (1997) hierarchy. It also coincides with Kerlinger's empirical knowledge. Empirics is organised systematically into scientific principles, theories and laws for the purpose of describing, explaining and predicting phenomena of special concern to nursing. The quantifiability of empirical data allows objective measurement that yields evidence that can be replicated by multiple observers (Carper 1992). We would argue that on occasions nurses can ignore this type of knowledge because it is superseded by one or more of Carper's other types of knowing.

Aesthetics

As you would gather from previous sections, empirics is a rather narrow perspective. Nursing practice may also be perceived as an art and Carper acknowledged this in the pattern of knowing called aesthetics. It gives us the knowledge that focuses on the craft of nursing that involves tacit knowledge, skill and intuition. It reflects Rhyl's 'know-how knowledge' and has its roots in the philosophy of historicism. Aesthetic knowledge is subjective, individual and unique. It enables us to go beyond that which is explained by existing laws and theories and to accept that there are phenomena that cannot be quantified. Therefore, intuition, interpretation, understanding and valuing make up the central components of aesthetics.

We could argue that armed with this *aesthetics* knowing, nurses could ignore *empirics* knowing. For instance, many research-based scales assess and predict patients' risk of pressure damage. Nonetheless, clinical judgement based on experience and intuition are also used. Similarly, research evidence may provide guidance on when patients can mobilise postoperatively, but the intuitive expertise of the nurse regarding the patient's ability may justifiably override this.

Ethics

Carper's third pattern of knowing is called ethics. This type of knowing provides us with knowledge that is about what is right and wrong and what is good and bad, desirable and undesirable. It is expressed through moral codes and ethical decision-making. In everyday practice nurses often have to make choices between competing interventions. These choices and judgements may have an ethical dimension and to select the most appropriate position or action requires careful deliberation. For example, for ethical reasons, some nurses may decide not to participate in a particular treatment even though the results from clinical trials or other studies (empirics) note that it is effective for some conditions. For example, we know of nurses who will not participate in electroconvulsive therapy or therapeutic abortions. Ethical evidence may also be used to make decisions about the costs and benefits of treatment in terms of quality-of-life years, or whether terminally ill people should be actively resuscitated.

Personal knowing

Like aesthetics, 'personal knowing' is subjective yet is about us being aware of ourselves and how we relate to others. It represents knowledge that focuses on self-consciousness, personal awareness and empathy. If, as various theorists argue, caring is an interpersonal process (Peplau 1995a) where interactions and transactions between people are central (King 1981), then we must know our own strengths and weaknesses in order to be expert practitioners. At our best we do not perceive patients as objects but instead have a genuine relationship with those requiring care. We can learn as much from a caring relationship as they do and a good caring relationship will depend on our own self-regard. Therefore, personal knowing requires self-consciousness and active empathic participation on the part of the knower (Carper 1992). Here again, the influence of historicism is evident.

It is possible that nurses may reject empirical evidence because of their personal knowing. For example, consider the situation where a nurse is working with a patient or a family member who is going through a grief reaction. Despite research findings that suggest a linear movement through a number of grieving stages, the nurse's personal experience may indicate that not everyone has to go through all these phases or in the order suggested by the empirical evidence.

Carper's work has undergone careful analysis by many authors (see Silva et al. 1995; Meleis 2007). Experienced nurses use these four patterns of knowing interchangeably. For instance, experienced oncology nurses will be aware of the research and theoretical basis for providing chemotherapy (empirics) and they have the skills and intuition to ensure the patient understands the treatment and is as comfortable as possible while receiving it (aesthetics). However, the issue of withholding chemotherapy because of severe side-effects and sometime poor prognosis is a moral decision to be made with the patient (ethics). Finally, knowing themselves and their inner resources is important in the construction of an interpersonal therapeutic relationship with the client (personal knowing).

As you reflect on these four patterns of knowing you will note the complexity of nursing knowledge. The patterns are not mutually exclusive; there is overlap, interrelation and interdependence. By recognising that there are legitimate ways of knowing other than empirical knowing, Carper has made a valuable contribution to the examination of knowledge development in nursing. Further, as outlined above, it may be possible to reject empirical knowing because of the influence of one or more of the other ways of knowing.

Chinn and Kramer (2004) stated that *empirics* removed from the context of the whole of knowing produces control and manipulation, removing *ethics* produces rigid doctrine and insensitivity to the rights of others, removing *aesthetics* produces prejudices, bigotry and lack of appreciation of meaning, and removing *personal knowing* produces isolation and self-distortion.

Activity 3: Frameworks for knowing

Earlier we noted Kerlinger's categories of knowledge, and above we note Carper's patterns of knowing.

Consider how each might help inform our study and practice of nursing. Do you think there may be something in one scheme that is missing in the other, and if so, how might the schemes be brought together?

Also, identify different clinical interventions that use all four of Carper's patterns of knowing.

Linking knowing with theory

Knowledge is of little use without understanding and understanding is gained by theory. It is a reciprocal relationship; while knowledge can increase in nursing for a time without understanding, understanding is not possible without new knowledge being developed. Theory has to keep pace with knowledge development; if not, stagnation of the discipline will occur.

Theory is overused and often abused in speech. People say: 'I have a theory as to why X is occurring' or 'in theory this should work' or 'theoretically, X is better than Y' or 'the theory is that you place Z here' or, a more familiar statement to nurses, 'the theory–practice gap is ruining the profession'. As a word, theory is common currency in ordinary conversation but it means different things to different people. People have different theories as to why President Kennedy was assassinated or why Princess Diana died. Regardless of its use as a term, you will detect that theory is about knowing or understanding.

To explore this further we wish to return in more detail to some work we referred to in Activity 3 in the previous chapter. In a landmark paper, two philosophers, James Dickoff and Patricia James (1968), identified four levels of theory for nursing. These are:

1 Factor-isolating theory: describes and names concepts.
2 Factor-relating theory: relates concepts to one another.
3 Situation-relating theory: interrelationship among concepts or propositions.
4 Situation-producing theory: prescribes actions to reach certain outcomes.

You will recall that they proposed two crucial arguments: first, in ascending order each of these levels builds on previous levels so factor-isolating theory is a precursor of factor-relating theory, and so on; second, a practice discipline like nursing requires situation-producing theory so that nurses could, with a degree of certainty, prescribe interventions that lead to desired outcomes for patients.

Earlier, we denigrated empiricists and positivists for being overly concerned with hierarchies. Here too we would point to the fact that Dickoff and James have introduced a hierarchy of theories in nursing. Furthermore, they stress that the highest level – situation-producing theory – is the most important for our discipline. This assertion may be true but it has the potential to place the other three levels in a lowly and less well-regarded location. We could of course argue that all four levels are very important because without the first three the final and most prestigious level cannot be achieved. This would not be the same with Muir Gray's (1997) hierarchy of evidence or Kerlinger's (1986) levels of knowing.

In Chapter 2, the differences between grand theory, middle range theory and practice theory were briefly outlined. In essence, Dickoff and James's situation-producing theory is practice theory by another name. They posited rightly that nursing is a practice discipline and therefore theory is needed that will allow nurses to know with a degree of certainty that if they do X, then Y will happen. You would agree that such knowledge and understanding is of crucial importance to any practice discipline.

Research as a basis for knowledge development

Research is defined as 'rigorous and systematic enquiry conducted on a scale and using methods commensurate with the issue to be investigated, and designed to lead to more generalised contributions to knowledge' (DoH 1994: 37). With its emphasis on generalisation it is possible in Department of Health terminology to see plainly the influence of positivism.

Nurses, in attempting to gain academic respect with other more long-established professions, adopted the positivist approach over other forms of enquiry when developing and testing theories (Suppe & Jacox 1985). Those nurses who pioneered other methods of enquiry, relating to understanding rather than control, were seldom given the recognition they deserved.

Nonetheless, the contribution of the positivistic research approach to nursing knowledge cannot be denied and it should not be rejected completely. In Britain there have been some very good research projects which, although having their basis in the experimental positivist tradition, have contributed substantially to nursing knowledge.

New methods of research do not just happen; they are the products of much philosophical thought and discussion. One broad approach was based on what Wilhelm Dilthey (1833–1911) referred to as 'human science'. Readers will note from the following that it emanates from the historicist philosophy of science.

Human science values subjective opinion, beliefs, personal knowledge, descriptions of experiences and feelings, much of which are not amenable to objective verification. Human science also recognises the effects that the researcher and the research participants/respondents have on what is being researched. Intuition, understanding, reflection, meanings and experiences are central components of the human science approach. Within human science the participants' 'lived experiences' are the core of explanations and meanings about things, and are interpreted by them, not by outsiders. Humans are perceived as whole people and breaking them down into components is dehumanising. Conversations and interactions require interpretation and uncovering patterns in these is an appropriate goal of human science.

Human science is often referred to as the *perceived view* as opposed to the *received view* of empiricism (Table 3.3).

Chinn and Kramer (2004) accepted the importance of both views for the development of knowledge for practice. In traditional science an attempt is made to study the whole through looking at its parts, while in human science an attempt is made to study the whole as it appears. In traditional science, knowledge is developed to describe, to explain and to predict; in human science, knowledge is developed to understand. In traditional science, theory is developed through defining, analysing and synthesising concepts and propositions; in human science, theory is developed through description and interpretation. Traditional science is directed towards uncovering cause-and-effect relationships and generalisations, human science is directed towards creating knowledge from common meanings, patterns and themes in descriptions. However, both seek empirical honesty through methodological rigour (Smith 1994: 51).

In contrast, Susan Gadow (1990) did not think human science went far enough in explaining how best to develop nursing knowledge. She believed that the researcher should leave the personal alone and experience alone because there is no way to summarise (reduce) a life, a culture or any human situation. Qualitative research is no better than quantitative here in that it treats experience as data. She appeared to argue that quantitative researchers may be more honest because they are 'up front' in calling the subject the object of their study (cited in Smith 1994).

Table 3.3 The received view versus the perceived view.

Received view	Perceived view
Objective	Subjective
Deduction	Induction
One truth	Multiple truths
Validation and replication	Trends and patterns
Justification	Discovery
Test theories	Evaluate theories
Prediction and control	Description and understanding
Particulars	Patterns
Reductionism	Holism
Generalisation	Individualism
Empirical positivism	Historicism

Nonetheless, it is heartening that nurses are beginning to accept and use methods of enquiry other than the empiricist approach to develop and test knowledge. This should have a powerful effect in identifying a body of knowledge that has particular relevance to patient care. In this way 'know-that' and 'know-why' knowledge can enrich the 'know-how' knowledge and vice versa.

Developing nursing knowledge through reasoning

Inductive reasoning

Every day, practitioners deal with client phenomena. By taking note of patterns and commonality in those phenomena that are of special interest to nursing, it is possible to build up a body of knowledge. This is referred to as inductive reasoning and it reflects moving from the specific to the general. The early empiricists favoured this method when developing theory. Qualitative research approaches from the historicist school of philosophy also use induction to generate theory (know-that knowledge) from practice (know-how knowledge).

Deductive reasoning

In contrast to inductive reasoning, deductive reasoning involves moving from the general to the specific. You will note elsewhere in this chapter that Rene Descartes favoured it as a key component of rationalism. Deductive reasoning traditionally involves the use of three propositions (two premises and one conclusion). In deductive reasoning a conclusion follows from one or more statements that are taken as true. Aristotle (384–322 BC) perfected this form of deductive argument calling it a syllogism (Stokes 2004). The most famous example is:

All men are mortal (1st premise) (axiom 1 or postulate 1);
Socrates is a man (2nd premise) (axiom 2 or postulate 2);
Therefore, Socrates is mortal (conclusion) (theorem).

Here the reasoning goes from the general (all men) to the specific (Socrates). You can see that if the premises remain the same but we changed the conclusion to read 'Socrates is not mortal' then the deductive reasoning would be faulty.

You could reverse the example and make it inductive reasoning. Here the reasoning goes from specifics (Confucius, Socrates, Hannibal) to the general (all men). So a series of discrete observations about phenomena are followed by a conclusion:

Confucius is a man and is mortal (1st premise);
Socrates is a man and is mortal (2nd premise);
Hannibal is a man and is mortal (3rd premise);
Therefore, all men are mortal (conclusion).

Deductive reasoning in nursing normally starts with an established theory and this (or part of it) is tested in the real world of practice to see if it can be disproved – remember our reference to Karl Popper's (1965) work on refutation.

Retroductive reasoning

Whether theories should be developed deductively or inductively is seen as a false argument by Jacox and Webster (1992). They state that some attempts will use a more deductive or a more inductive approach than others but all theory construction includes both. To them, it is not an either-or issue. This amalgamation of induction and deduction is referred to as retroduction. An example of this type of research would be that of Boore (1978). Boore used an experimental design to test the theory that providing information to preoperative patients would reduce their stress levels postoperatively. Since a specific theory was being tested and applied, the method used was deduction. However, the results of this study led to new practices in how patients are prepared for surgery and a 'practice theory' of preoperative preparation was developed. Here, Boore was using induction where experiences within the research setting led to the development of a new, more clinically specific, theory.

Summary

This chapter showed that there are many ways of knowing in nursing. It highlighted the main philosophies of science underpinning how and why people develop knowledge. The armchair rationalist approach to knowledge development popularised by Descartes was influential in its day but by the mid 18th century empiricists set down the rules that were to influence healthcare research ever since. Empiricism is still alive and well in nurses' use of randomised controlled trials, experiments and quasi-experiments. More recently, many nurse researchers have embraced phenomenology, an approach emanating from the tradition of historicism.

The importance of know-how, know-that and know-why knowledge was discussed and, while the strengths of each were highlighted, the need for nurses to know why is crucial for a practice discipline. This is reflected in Dickoff and James's fourth level of theory which provides nurses with the necessary ammunition to prescribe interventions that will have a positive effect on patients, their families and communities. However, Carper's work reminded us that there are other ways of knowing and her views are reflected in the differences between the received view and the perceived view.

There is a wealth of literature to suggest that nurses use several ways of knowing and that many of these do not fit neatly within the empirical framework. These patterns of knowing are being incorporated into contemporary theorising leading to new theoretical perspectives.

In conclusion, all types of knowing and knowledge development are valuable. Placing one in a higher position than another is not helpful; it depends on what knowledge is being sought and what questions are being addressed.

Nursing Theories and Nursing Roles

'It is a capital mistake to theorise before one has data.'
The Crooked Man, in *The Memoirs of Sherlock Holmes*,
Sir Arthur Conan Doyle (1859–1930)

Outline of content

The impact of worldwide advances in healthcare systems upon the roles of healthcare professionals is noted. In particular, the introduction of new and innovative roles to meet these new challenges is described. Particular attention is paid to the use of theory to inform practice in circumstances where methods of care delivery are changing, and where multidisciplinary approaches are being promoted.

Over recent years changes in health technology, professional knowledge and skills, and patient needs and expectations have made healthcare a dynamic area in which to work. The ageing population, the increase in chronic disease, the growth of day surgery, the expansion of primary care and the continued reduction in the length of hospital stay have all contributed to changing patterns of need and demand (Read et al. 2001).

These changes are occurring in healthcare systems throughout the world and are having an impact on the type of care provided and the format of its provision (Wilson et al. 2003). In particular, such changes have necessitated the development of new professional roles and practices (UKCC 2002). The new roles have brought with them a plethora of titles including specialist nurse practitioners, advanced nurse practitioners and nurse consultants. In many instances these roles incorporate practices which were previously undertaken by other professionals such as physicians, psychologists and social workers. The introduction of these new roles has been the topic of much debate in the literature (BMA 2002; Kendall & Lissauer 2003). However, the evidence base underpinning their introduction is limited (Buchan & Daz Pol 2002). There is also a dearth of knowledge as to whether or how the holders of these new roles use theory to inform their thinking and practice. Therefore, this chapter proposes to explore how role theory influences their development and practice and how nurses in new roles can use theories from a variety of disciplines to inform and improve care. It will also address whether grand theories, middle range theories or practice theories are the most appropriate for new role holders.

Role theory

While 'role' as a concept has a perceived meaning and is one of the most popular phenomena in the social sciences, Hinshaw (1978) noted that roles are consistently difficult to define and analyse due to their multidimensional nature. Perhaps the most common definition is that role is the set of prescriptions defining what the behaviour should be in a specific job. Therefore, a common theme is that role pertains to the behaviours of particular persons (Thomas & Biddle 1966). Role theory represents a collection of concepts and a variety of propositions in the form of hypothetical predictions of how people will perform in a given job, or under what circumstances certain types of behaviour can be expected (Conway 1978). Concepts within role theory include role norms, role set, role stress, role confusion, role overlap and role conflict.

Hamans (1966) described 'role norms' to be the ideas in the minds of members of a group that specify what they ought to do and what they are expected to do under given circumstances. There are role expectations held by members of the 'role set' which surround an individual and which exert pressures on them and their performance in a given situation (Kahn et al. 1966), the 'role set' being the role relationships held by virtue of occupying a particular social status (Merton 1966). For instance, a role set for a nurse would typically comprise nursing colleagues, other health professional colleagues, patients and representatives from their employing organisation.

The consideration of role can be seen to be of particular relevance to those involved in new roles in nursing. After all, the context in which they work is changing and therefore the perceptions and expectations of their role (both from themselves, other professionals and patients) are also changing.

Lambert and Lambert (2001) reviewed literature on role stress/role strain in nursing and noted the effect of the work environment (e.g. high job demands, little support from peers, lack of essential resources). Role stress is defined as a condition in which role obligations are vague, irritating, difficult, conflicting or impossible to meet (Hardy 1978).

Last and Self (1994) observed that for a number of years there had been discussion about the 'extended role' of the nurse with very little clarity about what 'extension' means. More recently, Daly and Carnwell (2003) noted that nursing practice is getting more diverse and the boundaries of inter- and intra-professional practices and competencies are becoming increasingly blurred. Halsey (1978) observed that nurse leaders must deal with role prescriptions from a variety of sources and often the demands and expectations of one group of people are inconsistent with those of other groups. Therefore, with the confusion surrounding role development and professional isolation, there is the potential for role stress among those who hold new roles in nursing.

Role conflict is defined as divergence between the role expectations among different members of the role set (Bower et al. 2004). Bower studied the introduction of a new primary healthcare role and concluded that the specification of the post holder in the new role and the expectations among existing staff increased the potential for role conflict. In Northern Ireland, McKenna et al. (2003) investigated professional and lay views in relation to generic and specialist roles in the community and noted that there was concern that specialisation (while welcome) would lead to role conflict, role overlap and role confusion. Pearson (2003) argued that role confusion and conflict have become endemic in nursing for a number of reasons. He concluded that although the contribution of nursing is difficult to define in an evolving profession, the re-thinking of role boundaries has never been as important as it is now. It is not surprising that Benner (1984) pointed out that role complexity and responsibility require long-term continuing development.

It is important to understand role theory in the context of new role developments in nursing. Two terms have been used to describe this phenomenon: role expansion and role extension. The former means that nurses retain their occupational focus but the work within the role expands. For example, if a nursing role is focused on health promotion, then widening the role in health promotion signifies role expansion. In contrast, role extension occurs when nurses extend their remit almost 'amoeba-like' into that of another discipline. So nurses taking on a prescribing remit or minor surgery would be undergoing role extension. This lends itself to role confusion, role overlap and role conflict. These occur at the boundary when doctors are shedding duties that were once entirely within their remit and when nurses are moving to take on these duties. If both parties do not come to the realisation at the same time, role conflict and confusion can occur. At such times, care quality and patient safety can be compromised (McKenna 2004).

Activity 1: The use of non-nursing theories to shed light

Thus far we have considered the meaning of the term 'role'. We have also recognised that it has certain dynamic attributes. You have been introduced to role theory which, like all theories, is composed of a number of concepts linked by statements called propositions. Some of these concepts include role expansion, role extension, role norms, role set, role stress, role confusion, role overlap and role conflict.

   You can see that a theory from the social sciences (role theory) can help describe, explain and possibly predict behaviour that is of importance in understanding nursing. We suggest that you visit the literature and identify another non-nursing theory that impacts on how nurses work. For example, you might focus on learning theory, the theory of planned action, or communication theory. Write a page about it including its main concepts and how these relate to each other. You could usefully discuss this with your fellow students.

Interagency/interprofessional changes

In recent years there has also been a drive towards more effective interprofessional working. The ENRiP (Exploring New Roles in Practice) study concluded that each profession would need to rethink its traditional recruitment, education, professional development and career patterns so that joint working is facilitated (Read et al. 2001). This also has implications for the use of theory. Practice underpinned by nursing theory may seem alien to other health professionals whereas borrowed or multidisciplinary theory lends itself well to interprofessional working.

   The future of nursing has been described as an investment in the quality of partnership, not only with the patient, but also the rest of the healthcare team (Castledine 2003). Further, the development of new nursing roles, especially into the medical field, will not be achieved safely without co-operation between the different disciplines (Rose et al. 1997). The increasing reliance on non-registered staff (healthcare assistants) to deliver care under the supervision of qualified professionals has also been a factor affecting role overlap and role confusion among interprofessional care teams (Bridges et al. 2003). This can also lead to theory overlap and theoretical confusion. For example, within oncology a medical model focusing on cure could conflict with a nursing model based on care and palliation. These conflicting approaches have the potential to confuse patients and their families.

Confusion surrounding innovative roles

Rose et al. (1997) stated that despite much debate, the questions about the nature, scope and professional autonomy of nurses as clinical practitioners have yet to be clarified. The range of titles used by those occupying new roles does not help. Barnes (2004) stressed that the confusion surrounding nursing titles extended beyond patients to other health professionals associated with nursing, and to nurses themselves. This is not a new concern; the Scottish Office (SODH 1995) maintained that the different academic requirements for specialist and advanced practitioner posts caused perplexity. Similarly, the Welsh Institute for Health and Social Care (WIHSC 2004) noted the wide range of titles in use among post-registration nurses and stressed the importance of ensuring that the public was able to understand the learning that underpins these titles. McKenna et al. (2005) found the same concerns in Northern Ireland.

According to Castledine (2003) many of the first nurse specialist roles developed without clear direction or control. Their unstructured emergence appeared to be linked to individual medical consultants and was often confined to specialist areas (Cameron & Masterson 2000). Earlier, Levenson and Vaughan (1999) designed a guide for those setting up new roles (developed from the ENRiP project). They asserted that the first key issue is clarity about the purpose and function of the role. Both of these are influenced by the theoretical orientation within the role. For instance, if a nurse adheres to Orem's self-care theory (Orem 1980, 1985, 1995), the purpose and function of her role will reflect that orientation. In contrast, if Henderson's activities of living (Henderson 1966) is the theory used, the purpose and function will differ.

Bridges et al. (2003) used an action research approach to explore the impact of one new role (interprofessional care co-ordinators) in a large London trust. They noted that the tensions arising with this new role were associated with the lack of fit of the role within the hospital's traditional hierarchy. This lack of fit within existing structures was also found in a Northern Ireland evaluation of an oncology nurse specialist role (McKenna et al. 2004). In the latter case the nurse's theoretical orientation on compassion and care conflicted with the physician's emphasis on technology and cure.

The Scope of Professional Practice (UKCC 1992: 1) stated that nurses must be 'sensitive, relevant and responsive to the needs of individual patients . . . and have the capacity to adjust when and where to changing circumstances'. This emphasises theories of human need (e.g. Minshull et al. 1986). While this provides a rationale for role function and development, it also indicates that the responsibility for defining the scope of practice of the advanced role will be determined by the individual practitioner (Denner 1995).

Accountability

Accountability for the scope of new roles and the standards of practice that apply to them are often unclear. Semple and Cable (2003) maintained that accountability involves taking personal responsibility for actions and no individual can be accountable for another. If things go wrong, practitioners may be at risk of complaints and disciplinary or legal action as a result of the groundbreaking innovatory nature of their work and the lack of clear guidance on accountability. Rose et al. (1997) debated whether nurses should consider their ability to defend themselves legally before agreeing to extend their scope of practice.

The issues concerning the accountability and responsibility accepted by innovative role post holders have included discussion on the use of theories, protocols and guidelines. If the role is truly innovative, then rigid adherence to older theories could stifle creativity. The same applies to the potentially protective function of evidence-based protocols, with some viewing them as too restrictive. Theories, guidelines and protocols do not have the force of statutory regulation and Rose et al. (1997) considered that there is room for discussion on whether patients' interests would be best served if they were used to underpin all new innovative roles.

Isolation and burnout

Scholes et al. (1999) suggested that innovative roles can lead to isolation and 'burnout', especially when there is minimal support within the organisation. The support of managers is a critical factor for the successful transition to new roles. The innovative nature of some roles can also mean that accessibility to colleagues in similar roles is difficult. This suggests that there are limited opportunities to discuss professional and practice issues, or identify possible mentors. Furthermore, colleagues may fail to understand the post holders' skills and contribution (Davies 2001). McKenna et al. (2005) found that linking with colleagues who shared similar jobs and theoretical perspectives was important for personal and professional identity, as well as providing a resource for support and debriefing. However, if different diabetic nurse specialists used different theories to inform their practice, this could encourage isolation and a lack of sharing best practice.

Inconsistency in role development

In the UK, Buchan and Seccombe (2003) highlighted a range of initiatives to encourage team working, develop advanced roles, support the introduction of different skill mixes and encourage flexible working. In addition, a wide range of UK courses and programmes to support specialist practice have developed. However, there have been regional differences in funding the training required to prepare practitioners for new roles, with inequitable access to courses.

Local policies have created inconsistencies in role development and may therefore lead to a clash between personal and professional values. There may also be regional variation in the number and type of specialist nurses, particularly in more remote and rural areas. Once again this is accentuated by the use of different theories by different specialist and advanced nurses in different parts of the country.

Further, there is a question on how nurse educators should teach nursing theory to specialist and advanced nurses. Should they restrict their curriculum content to one or two theories or should they present dozens of theories to students? While the former approach is restricting, it does encourage understanding and collaboration between practitioners and across clinical settings. In contrast, the latter approach encourages greater theoretical sophistication but has the potential to confuse and restrict communication between practitioners and settings.

Deskilling of generalist practitioners

The generalist versus the specialist debate has been ongoing in the nursing literature (McKenna et al. 2003). The potential deskilling of the 'generalist' nurse has also been highlighted as a concern for those debating the role of the specialist nurse. Interestingly, specialist nurses may want to keep specialist knowledge to themselves and generalist nurses may be happy to leave complex issues of patient care to their specialist colleagues.

McGee and Castledine (1999) studied the expectations of senior personnel in 371 trusts in England (response rate 62%, $n = 230$). Fifty of the respondents argued that the employment of specialist nurses could result in the deskilling of other staff (doctors as well as nurses). There was also concern that nurses could become too focused on a specialty and this could lead to professional isolation and a loss of generic skills. Jack et al. (2004) found this potential deskilling of ward nurses being voiced by student nurses. The cause for this was the generalist being said to 'pass the buck' to the specialist and the specialist being said to 'adopt a sense of superiority' to the generalist. It is also possible that the more talented and qualified nurses are those who are 'creamed off' to the specialist roles and that this could be to the detriment of the remaining staff and may result in a deterioration of standards and outcomes.

It is also the case that specialist nurses are more likely to use middle range theories (Merton 1966) while generalist nurses will use broader grand theories. This is understandable but it could lead to an added barrier to communication between generalists and specialists. You can predict that employing different middle range and grand theories will encourage the use of conceptual language that is not shared across the generalist–specialist divide.

Influence of the medical model on nursing roles

Put simply, the medical model is composed of concepts such as assessment, diagnosis, prescription and treatment. It is the theoretical framework used by most doctors in their everyday practice. For many years nurses have been berated for basing their teaching and practice on this model.

The medical model has a long history and it is no surprise that it has influenced the development of some nursing roles and been the impediment of others. Florence Nightingale (1859) was of the opinion that medicine and nursing roles should be clearly differentiated from each other. Prior to the establishment of her nurse training school at St Thomas's Hospital in London, nurses were lower-order 'Sairey Gamp'-like figures. In contrast, physicians came from the respectable middle and upper middle classes and, inevitably, their social and educational backgrounds were very different from those of the nurses who were their subordinates. Therefore, in Nightingale's 19th century, doctors and nurses were separated by their gender, social class, language and education. This differentiation was to remain for most of the 20th century.

The scientific basis for the medical model can be traced back to Hippocrates, Aristotle and Galen. From Chapter 3, readers will recall that in the early 17th century Descartes fostered the notion of the body as a machine. Disease was viewed as the consequence of breakdown and the physician's task was to repair the machine. Most physicians base their treatment philosophy on this fundamental tenet of reductionism. This implies that all behavioural phenomena must be conceptualised in terms of physiochemical principles (Engel 1977). Over the years this basic precept has been accepted not only by many healthcare professionals but also by the public.

Within the medical model the preliminary assessment is of great importance to physicians. The initial examination will ultimately lead to the recognition of signs and symptoms. Kim (1989) believed that the proponents of the medical model have a vested interest in searching for abnormal clinical features to confirm the presence of illness. These signs and symptoms are categorised into patterns which in turn form the basis for diagnostic labelling. Chapman (1985) maintained that such labelling has a dehumanising effect because the client is envisaged as little more than a disease entity.

For the medical model, knowing the disease inevitably determines the treatment strategy. The goals of therapy are seldom client centred, and the individual must assume the client role with the concomitant obligation to co-operate (McKenna 1990). This compliance is an important element in the treatment process. Traditionally, nurses were expected to comply and co-operate with the physician's orders. They were discouraged from providing information to the patient about their possible prognosis – this was the doctor's job. Therefore, while the therapeutic plan may present the facade of an egalitarian team approach, the doctor as the healer was viewed as superior to all other health professionals.

Due to the traditional hierarchy within healthcare, nurses were subservient within a handmaiden role (Aggleton & Chalmers 2000). This servile position was seen by many to be due to our tenacious reliance on the medical model (Meave 1994). According to Peplau, 'Well into the 1940s, many textbooks for nurses, often written by physicians, clergy, or psychologists reminded nurses that theory was too much for them, that nurses did not need to think but rather merely to follow rules, be obedient, be compassionate, do their duty, and carry out medical orders' (Peplau 1987: 18).

According to Stockwell (1985), as an observer of signs and symptoms, the nurse was the eyes and ears of the doctor, and as a practitioner she was his hands and feet, carrying out the prescribed treatment. Having such a single role focus does not allow for independent action and there was a danger that it may lead practitioners to ignore aspects of the client which do not fit neatly within the boundaries of the medical model. Constrained within this model, nurses were ill equipped to care for the patient as a whole person or the family as a whole unit.

Because of intense scrutiny by nurse theorists, the limitations of the medical model soon became apparent. Paramount among these was the 'sick role'. Parsons (1952) recognised that patients, as exemplified by the sick role, had the right to be relieved from social roles and the right not to be held responsible for their illness or condition. They are, however, obliged to seek professional help and to try their best to get well. This diverts attention away from potentially important social and psychological factors, which have little currency within the medical model. One person differing from another in terms of race, sex, age, marital status, religion or social class is merely an item for the briefest consideration.

Nursing's adherence to physicians' orders fostered a fascination with cure, with care often being placed in a secondary position. It is no surprise that when faced with illness, members of the public value the emphasis on cure. However, cure without care is an empty phenomenon and many chronic and terminal illnesses require an emphasis on care and palliation rather than cure.

The reduction in junior doctors' working hours through the European Working Time Directive has led managers to realise that there will not be enough junior doctors to fulfil the requirement of a hard-pressed health service. There are three options: train and employ more doctors, train and employ doctor's assistants, or encourage nurses to take on more medical roles. The latter is the cheapest and quickest option and in the early 21st century more and more duties that were once the sole responsibility of physicians are being undertaken by nurses. In turn, nurses may transfer much of their 'basic nursing care' to untrained assistants. Like the allied health professionals, nursing is in a state of flux, trying to decide whether to embrace physicians' roles or retain the traditional roles. We would offer a note of caution: nurses must ensure that slavishly following the medical agenda does not leave them in a type of 'limbo' between caring and curing.

More recently, concern has been expressed over the development of new nursing roles in areas that were previously the remit of medicine. It has been concluded that one of the ways in which roles were developed was on a medical substitution basis (Scholes et al. 1999; Scholes & Vaughan 2002). Ewens (2003) stated that this development is attractive to a profession like nursing, which has been dogged by insecurity, low status and gender inequality. Previously, Rose et al. (1997) argued that it is not acceptable for nurses to undertake medical work at the expense of nursing work. Castledine (2003) supported this stance, asserting that there is a danger of the nurse specialist following a medicalised descriptor of his or her role. This is due, in part, to the failure of the nursing profession in defining not only specialist nursing, but generalist nursing practice.

For instance, we are aware of nurses whose entire working day is spent removing veins from patients' legs. These veins are later used by surgeons in heart bypass operations. These nurses are well paid and well trained for this role but we suggest that, as an example of role extension, it should not be classed as a nursing role or as a means of developing nursing as a profession.

It is a given that due to new technologies, knowledge and skills in all professions progress to new practices, leaving behind what may be perceived as mundane tasks and duties. After all, to remain professionally static is to go backwards. Accepting this, nurses have to be careful with regard to what they shed from their professional portfolio. If they unthinkingly take on more medical work they could become little more than technicians and in the process transfer to unqualified assistants those practices that patients and their families value most highly. If nurses become 'mini-doctors' will they have a greater affiliation to the medical model or will they bring with them the best aspects of nursing theories?

The medical model has major advantages for the treatment of illness. Advances in medically oriented cures have freed many clients from the effects of disturbing symptomatology and contributed to their early discharge. Mitchell (1986) believed that because of the medical model's universality, prospective clients are familiar with it and as a result the public find it comforting to be cared for within a framework they can recognise.

Activity 2: Exploring the medical model

As will be noted above, the so-called medical model may emphasise certain attributes that nurses view negatively (a very instrumental and depersonalised approach, a concern with cases rather than people, and with pathology rather than person, etc.). However, it was noted that the model also had some positive or redeeming attributes.

Undertake a brief review of the literature and seek to identify at least three positive and three negative aspects of the medical model.

Return to Chapter 2, and under the section on 'Practical knowledge as sophisticated knowledge' re-read the passages on gnostic and pathic touch. Consider how the ideas expressed there help to clarify the differences between medicine and nursing. Reflect upon how these two methods of touching may be important in nursing *and* medicine.

It is important that nurses in new roles take cognisance of these factors and realise the imprudence of rejecting the medical model in its entirety. Within any nursing theory the biological and pathological perspective of the individual must be respected. Nonetheless, nursing's disenchantment with the pervasiveness of the medical model has been one of the main reasons for the development of theories in nursing. Now that nurses are bringing their unique perspective to the job, the medical model no longer suffices.

You will recall from Chapters 2 and 3 that there are three main levels of theory. We also intimated that metatheory is sometimes referred to as a fourth level. Nonetheless for this section we will focus on the three levels that in part reflect Merton's (1966) categorisations:

1   Grand theory
2   Middle range theory
3   Practice theory.

We will argue that grand theory has limited value for those nurses who have taken on new roles. In contrast, the less abstract and more easily operationalised middle range and practice theories have become crucially important for such nurses.

Relevance of existing 'grand' nursing theories

McKenna (1997) estimated that there are over 50 nursing theories. However, most of these were formulated many decades ago. The obvious point to consider is whether these old theories are still relevant for the new roles that nurses are undertaking or whether there is a need for their adaptation or their amalgamation with the medical model.

Hildegard Peplau (1952) has been given credit for formulating the first contemporary theory in nursing. After leaving Columbia University she developed her theory inductively through reflecting on a long career in psychiatric nursing. She also developed it deductively through the influence of Harry Stack Sullivan's (1953) interpersonal relations theory. Peplau's work influenced later theorists who used 'interpersonal relationships' as a basis for their work, i.e. Henderson (Henderson & Harmer 1955), Orem (1959), Johnson (1959) and Hall (1959).

The 1960s saw the publication of theories by Abdellah (Abdellah et al. 1960), Orlando (1961), Wiedenbach (1964), Levine (1966), Travelbee (1966) and King (1968). Of these, Abdellah, Orlando and Travelbee were undoubtedly influenced by Peplau. We would argue that many of the new roles undertaken by nurses require expertise in interpersonal relationships. After all, specialist nurses are the lead practitioners for a range of services such as diabetes clinics, health promotion clinics and clinics for adults with depression.

In the mid 1960s, Henderson, Wiedenbach and Orlando, previously students at Columbia University in New York, obtained employment as lecturers in the Yale School of Nursing. Here, theorists began to study how nurses practised and the effect this had on patients. Myra Levine, while also working at Yale, put forward her conservational theory of nursing (Levine 1966). It was also at Yale that the philosophers Dickoff and James (1968) wrote their seminal work on a 'theory of theories', referred to in Chapter 3. Their work led nurses to realise that they, as practitioners, could make a major contribution to the formulation and use of theory.

The rapid growth in the number of nursing theories witnessed in the 1960s continued into the 1970s, with the work of Roy (1970), Rogers (1970), Neuman (Neuman & Young 1972), Riehl (1974), Adam (1975), Patterson and Zderad (1976), Leininger (1978), Watson (1973, 1979) and Newman (1979). Unfortunately, many of the theorists simply presented their theory to the nursing masses and made no effort to critique, analyse or evaluate their work. Theorists were lauded across the US nursing fraternity and dissent against the new theories was discouraged.

While the 1980s witnessed an acceptance of the significance of theories for our discipline, in North America at least, there seemed to be a slowing down in the number of theories being developed. There, only three new nursing theories were published in the 1980s: the work of Parse (1981), Fitzpatrick (1982) and Erickson et al. (1983). Interestingly, Parse and Fitzpatrick constructed their theories not from first principles but from Martha Rogers's earlier theory (1970). This 'borrowing' of theory from other nurse theorists represented a new and interesting departure for the development of nursing knowledge.

While there was a slowing down in the development of new theories in the US, there was a surge in theory development in the UK. Although Nightingale's teachings are held up to be the first attempts at nurse theorising, the UK did not boast a pedigree of theory development. It was not until the 1980s and 1990s that some British nurses followed their American counterparts and began to formulate theories. Included in this is the work of Roper et al. (1983), McFarlane (1982), Stockwell (1985), Wright (1986), Castledine (1986), Clark (1986), Minshull et al. (1986), Green (1988), Bogdanovic (1989), Friend (1990), Yoo (1991) and Slevin (1995).

Most of these UK and US grand theories in nursing have been tried but not tested. Their broad scope and nebulousness has left many nurses disenchanted with them. While their philosophical underpinnings of self-care, interpersonal relationships, adaptation and interaction are still important for nurses, their inability to be operationalised has been a frustrating element and their use as frameworks to develop and lead practice has diminished in the late 20th and early 21st centuries.

Looking at grand theories through a 21st-century lens it can be argued that these theories were designed for a different era and a different type of nurse. Just as nurse teachers often castigate nursing students for using old literature, we too should question whether using nursing theories developed 40 or 50 years ago is appropriate when nursing has moved on philosophically and practically. It could be argued that we need new theories to reflect the multiple new roles that nurses are undertaking. Although nursing has extended its remit into medicine, the medical model may not serve nurses well in the brave new world that is specialist and advanced practice.

Relevance of existing 'middle range' nursing theories

In the 1990s and in the early years of the 21st century there appeared to be a move away from the 'grand theories' to 'middle range' theories. As alluded to above, grand theories are broad and abstract and do not easily lend themselves to application or testing. In contrast, middle range theories are moderately abstract and inclusive but are composed of concepts and propositions that are more testable. At their best, middle range theories balance the need for precision with the need to be sufficiently abstract (Merton 1968). They have fewer concepts and variables within their structure, are presented in a more testable form, have a more limited scope and have a stronger relationship with research and practice.

Merton (1968) maintained that middle range theories were particularly important for practice disciplines. This is of great relevance in the development of new roles. Specialist and advanced nurses require theories that are research based and can be operationalised in the delivery and enhancement of patient care. Although only recently receiving increasing attention in the UK, over 20 years ago there was a call for the development of middle range theories concerning the management of pain and the promotion of sleep (Jacox 1974). In the UK, the time is right for the development and employment of middle range theories by nurses in new roles.

Middle range theory tends to focus on concepts of interest to nurses. As well as pain, these include empathy, grief, self-esteem, hope, comfort, dignity and quality of life. Middle range theory can also grow from concept analysis (Cutcliffe & McKenna 2005). They help to close both the theory–practice and the research–practice gaps and to provide knowledge which is more readily applicable in direct care situations. Readers are referred to the middle range theory of comfort formulated by Katharine Kolcaba (2001) or to the maternal role attainment formulated by Ramona Mercer (1995).

Some middle range theories have their basis in grand theories. For example, the middle range theory of 'self-care deficit' grew out of Orem's (1980) grand theory of 'self care'. This supports Smith's assertion (1994) that a major function of grand theories is to act as a source for middle range theory. However, other middle range theories emerge from practice. For example, Swanson's (1991) middle range theory of 'caring in perinatal nursing' was inductively developed from studies in three perinatal settings. Similarly, Mishel (1990) developed a middle range theory of 'uncertainty' among patients. There are other middle range theories on menstrual care, family care-giving, relapse among ex-smokers, uncertainty in illness, perimenopausal process, self-transcendence, personal risk taking and illness trajectory. The beauty of middle range theories is that they can be applied readily to practice. From the foregoing literature it has been stressed that nurses in new roles are often professionally isolated (McKenna et al. 2005). Middle range theories can provide them with the theoretical and professional security that autonomy and accountability in new roles require. Nonetheless, cognisance should be taken of the threat they pose to communication and collaboration between generalist and specialist nurses and across different specialties.

Activity 3: From grand theory, to middle range theory to practice interface

It is suggested that grand theory (referred to earlier) is the higher-level framework from which mid-term theory derives. It is further suggested that middle range theories are typically specific enough to allow concrete issues or questions to be raised and then tested and applied within practice theory. This suggests that, in turn, practice theory is derived from middle range theory.

Carry out a brief literature review of the three forms of theory, concentrating mainly on the relationships between them. It is often difficult to explain such relationships in words. On this occasion, make notes during your review, but use these to produce a figure or diagram showing the relationships between the three forms.

Relevance of existing practice theories

Practice theories are very specific in their clinical focus and compared to middle range theory they are narrower in scope and more concrete in their level of abstraction. Jacox defined 'practice theory' as 'a theory that says – given this nursing goal (producing some desired change or effect in the patient's condition), these are the actions the nurse must take to meet the goal (produce the change)' (Jacox 1974: 10). From Chapters 2 and 3 you will note that these relate to Dickoff and James's (1968) highest level of theory.

Ten years earlier, Wald and Leonard (1964) were the first to argue for a 'practice theory' to guide nursing actions. They maintained that theory should emanate from practice and be used and tested in practice and have incorporated within it causal hypotheses. In other words, with practice theory a nurse should be able to say 'if I do this then the following will happen'. Therefore, practice theory prescribes the clinical interventions of the practising nurse.

The view of practice theory being a directive for practice is important for nurses in new roles. For instance, specialist nurses running a pain clinic know that they can reduce the patient's experience of pain by undertaking specific actions and nurses specialising in care of the elderly know that pressure area damage can be reduced by regular turning. Similarly, specialist preoperative nurses know that postoperative anxiety can be reduced by providing the patient with information before surgery. Because this may not happen every time with every patient, this is not a law; however, since it should have the desired effect with most patients, it represents practice theory. By using practice theory, nurses are going further than simply describing, explaining or predicting a phenomenon, they are prescribing actions that all being equal will have positive effects.

More so than middle range theory, practice theory provides the specialist or advanced practitioner with a repertoire of practices whereby the outcome is almost predictable. Wooldridge (1992) maintained that:

- Practice theory should be stated in such a way that the assumed cause–effect relationship between the mean(s) and the goals can be empirically tested.
- Practice theory should focus on causal agencies that are manipulable by the practitioner, on effects that are deemed relevant to evaluating the achievement of practice goals, and on those contingent conditions that are applicable to practice situations.
- Practice theories developed by a given profession should focus on the means for which that profession can assume autonomous prescriptive authority, both through direct manipulation of practice and the structuring of practice guidelines.

Summary

The number of new roles in nursing is increasing worldwide. In many cases these roles were previously the bailiwick of other health professionals. These new roles are having a major impact on nurses and nursing. To understand the issues it is important to understand role theory. This will illustrate for us the dangers of role strain, role confusion and role conflict.

Within these new roles nurses still require theories to guide their practice but there has been little discussion in the literature to help specialist nurse practitioners, advanced nurse practitioners or nurse consultants with theory selection. Because many of the new nursing roles were held previously by physicians it is unclear if the medical model should be embraced. Also, nursing theories that were formulated many decades ago may not be appropriate. These include most of the grand theories of the late 20th century. It is argued that the middle range theories and practice theories are most useful and these should be adopted as guides for prescribing nursing interventions.

Nursing Theories or Nursing Models?

'The use of nursing theories helps to make explicit to other professional groups that there is something called nursing which has an identity of its own, distinct from other similar activities . . . this would be a tremendous leap forward in the development of nursing as a profession.'

Smith (1982: 118)

Outline of content

The previous chapter described how new nursing roles and nursing theories have evolved and the importance of middle range and practice theories for guiding practice within these new roles. This chapter will further explain the often controversial relationship between theories and models and show how models can lead to the development of theory. In the following section it is proposed to examine these terms in detail and then compare and contrast them. The chapter will end by outlining the advantages and disadvantages of nursing theories.

Models

Some of the simplest definitions of a model describe it as a representation of reality (McFarlane 1986) or a simplified way of organising a complex phenomenon (Stockwell 1985). Other authors have elaborated on both these descriptions. Fawcett (2006) stated that a model is a set of concepts and the assumptions that integrate them into a meaningful configuration. Previously, Rambo (1984) asserted that a model was a way of representing a situation in logical terms to show the structure of the original idea or object.

McKenna (1994) has described a model as 'a mental or diagrammatic representation of care which is systematically constructed and which assists practitioners in organising their thinking about what they do, and in the transfer of their thinking into practice for the benefit of the patient and the profession'. Models therefore can be seen as conceptual tools or devices that can be used by an individual to understand and place complex phenomena into perspective.

Models take various forms: some models are presented in a one-dimensional format where they take the form of verbal statements or philosophical beliefs about phenomena. One-dimensional models tend to be at a high level of abstraction. They cannot be taken apart or explicitly observed, but they can be thought about and mentally manipulated.

Two-dimensional models include diagrams, drawings, graphs or pictures. Examples of such models include a diagram showing how to put together a piece of self-assembly furniture, the route map of London's underground rail network, and a diagrammatic representation of amino acid chains. Most models tend to begin as a one-dimensional conceptualisation and later develop into a two-dimensional format.

Three-dimensional models are what Craig (1980) referred to as physical models. These are scale models or structural replicas of things. In this form they may be intimately examined and manipulated. Examples of three-dimensional models include model toys, architectural scale models and anatomical models.

All three classes of model yield an enormous amount of information to those who use them. They tend to give a structured view of the particular circumstances under consideration. In this way the user is able to understand the represented concepts and the relationship of those concepts to each other.

Activity 1: The three model dimensions

Think of an object and conceptualise it using all three dimensions described above. For instance, you could take the example of a bodily organ. If you describe what it is and what it does, that is a one-dimensional model. Then draw a rough diagram of the organ, making it a two-dimensional model. This model may provide you with more information than the one-dimensional version. You could then obtain a plastic teaching replica of the organ in your school of nursing that can be taken apart and the internal structures manipulated. This three-dimensional model gives even more information about the structure of the organ than the previous two models.

You could do the same exercise with a kitchen appliance, a means of transport, and so on. Now that you get the idea, carry out the exercise and write a short note about the different dimensions and whether they gave you an increasing knowledge about the object.

Models have been employed in all fields of scientific enquiry. Their function is the same regardless of professional origin. They seek to clarify and elucidate. Mathematicians have used models for this purpose for thousands of years. In biology, Watson and Crick, who discovered the structure of the DNA helix, postponed celebrations and publication until after they had constructed a model.

Theories

One definition of theory is:

> 'a set of concepts, definitions and propositions that projects a systematic view of phenomena by designating specific interrelationships among concepts for the purpose of describing, explaining, predicting and/or controlling phenomena.' (Chinn & Kramer 2004: 70)

Other definitions of theory have been presented in earlier chapters. The following discussion will attempt to address the confusion that exists between models and theories.

Hildegard Peplau referred to her work as 'a set of concepts, a framework that can be applied to various kinds of nursing situations, but to call it a theory, I wouldn't' (cited in Suppe & Jacox 1985: 243). Nevertheless, Stevens Barnum (1998) viewed Peplau's formulations as a theory while Riehl and Roy (1974, 1980) called it a conceptual model. More recently, Peplau (1995a) did indeed refer to her work as a theory.

Similarly, Callista Roy's work (1971) was seen as a conceptual framework by Williams (1979), a grand theory by Kim (1983), an ideology by Beckstrand (1980) and as neither a model nor a theory by Webb (1986).

Dorothea Orem's conceptualisations (1980) have also been the object of some semantic confusion. Suppe and Jacox (1985) believed Orem had constructed a conceptual framework, Johnson (1983) preferred to view it as a descriptive theory, Rosenbaum (1986) favoured the title macro-theory, and the Nursing Theories Conference Group (George 1985) recognise it as a conceptual model.

Notwithstanding these contrary opinions, it is accepted by some authors that models are the most appropriate precursors of theory (Chinn & Kramer 1995; Fawcett 1995). This stance centres on their belief in the rigid criteria necessary for theory recognition, and the inability of many models to meet them. In essence, their position is that models are believed to lead to the identification of concepts and assumptions which, when tested by research, will ultimately lead to the formation of theory.

According to Fawcett (2005) models are more abstract than their theoretical counterparts. They present a generalised broader and abstract view of phenomena. Theories, on the other hand, are more specific and precise, containing more clearly defined concepts with a narrower focus. Therefore, the difference is one of abstraction, explication and application. We will refer to this argument as position A (see Figure 5.1).

This would appear to clear up any confusion. But taking a different stance to that of Fawcett, a group of metatheorists ably represented by Afaf Meleis (2007) and Barbara Stevens Barnum (1998) argued that it matters little what we call these things. They believe that much time has been wasted debating what the differences are between models, theories and paradigms. Rather, they maintain, time would be better spent evaluating the effects of these conceptualisations on patient care.

Meleis and Stevens Barnum base their argument on their desire to concentrate on content and not on labels. They asserted that theory

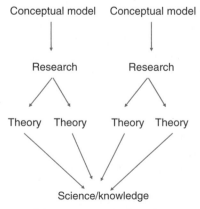

Figure 5.1 The theory–model controversy: Position A.

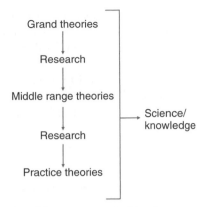

Figure 5.2 The theory–model controversy: Position B.

exists at different stages of development, from the most primitive to the most sophisticated form, and therefore even the simplest formulation is a theory. Their stance would be that models are theories but at a more abstract level than those theories developed through research. The former may be referred to as grand (or broad) theories while the latter are referred to as middle range or practice theories. We will refer to this view as position B (see Figure 5.2).

Activity 2: Position A or position B?

Both these positions can be supported by referring to various bodies of literature. We would urge you to view both approaches as worthy of consideration. However, for the purposes of this exercise, consider which position you are attracted to. Write down the pros and cons of each and your justification for selecting your favoured position.

See if this view concurs with that of other students. Check if they have identified the same or different advantages and disadvantages.

However, for the purpose of this book the term used to denote the conceptualisations put forward in the literature will be theories (position B). The basis for this decision lies with Meleis's call for professionals to concentrate on substance (content), not structure (terminology). When theories are mentioned in the remainder of this book, we will be referring to grand theories unless otherwise specified.

Accepting position B, it can be stated that theorists throughout the world have formulated approximately 50 grand theories which focus on nursing. Although many of these are referred to as nursing theories they are being used in midwifery practice. In Northern Ireland, for instance, Orem's self-care theory is used in many midwifery settings. This is reflected elsewhere. In 1988 Midgely surveyed 135 midwifery training schools and found that while 70 did not encourage the use of such theories, 24 of those that did used Orem's work.

As you saw from the previous chapter, twelve of the grand theories that do exist are British in origin while most of the rest emanated from North America.

Activity 3: Reasons for the evolution of theories

In Chapter 4 you saw a large list of theories that were developed in the USA and a shorter list ($n = 12$) of those developed in the UK. Form a small group with your fellow students and consider possible reasons why these theories were developed at those times and places.

Also, consider the reasons why there was a slowing down in the development of nursing theories in the US in the 1980s.

There are a number of possible answers to this issue. We include a sample to explain why theorising took place in 1950s America:

1 Disagreement with the medical model as a proper focus for our discipline.
2 The desire to develop a scientific basis for our practice.
3 The quest for professional recognition.
4 The advent of university education for nurses.
5 The increase in the number of masters/doctoral prepared nurses.
6 Women's contribution to the World War Two effort leading to an increase in questioning the female role in work and education.

We believe that the reasons why the number of new nursing theories decreased in 1980s America include the following. Many of the theorists began revising their work and examining how the status of middle range theory could be achieved. Interestingly, in the 1960s and 1970s several theorists were reluctant to claim theoretical status for their work. Perhaps such reluctance was not as widespread in the 1980s and 1990s. For example, King (1968) outlined her 'conceptual frame of reference'. However in her 1971 book, she appeared to be heading 'toward a theory for nursing', which when revised in 1981 was entitled *A Theory of Nursing*. This pattern of theoretical momentum is also evident in the writings of other theorists (Watson 1979, 1985; Parse 1981).

As was pointed out in Chapter 4, new 1980s theorists such as Parse (1981) and Fitzpatrick (Fitzpatrick & Whall 1983) built their work on

Martha Rogers's earlier theory (1970). It was commonplace for previous nurse theorists to use theories from other disciplines as a template for their work. However, this pattern of nurse theorists building on a previous nursing theory was a new and unique approach to theory development.

The stimuli for the development of theories in the UK in the 1980s just when nurse theorising was slowing down in the USA are interesting. It may have been the perception that American theories were not suitable for practice in the UK. Further, the introduction in the UK of higher education for nurses in the late 1970s forced many lecturers and students to look at how knowledge unique to these disciplines might be developed and taught on this side of the Atlantic. A similar trend can be seen in other countries of Europe and in Australia, where nursing programmes are being delivered within universities. In addition, as happened previously with their American counterparts, UK nurses began to examine the medical model and found it an inappropriate framework to guide nursing care.

Classification of theories

Since the mid 1970s there have been various attempts to categorise the large number of grand theories into a number of common types. Aggleton and Chalmers (2000) believed that this trend would help nurses make some preliminary decisions about the choice of theory that was most appropriate to a particular clinical setting. This grouping of theories by some trait also leads to an understanding of the various schools of thought that underpin each theory.

Often systems of cataloguing theories arise when editors of a book try to arrange them into some orderly scheme. For example, Meleis (2007) organised theories into those that describe what we do, those that describe how we do it, and those that describe the why of practice. In contrast, Stevens Barnum (1998) used the following classifications: intervention, conservation, substitution, sustenance and enhancement. Alligood and Marriner Tomey (2006) sorted theories into humanistic, interpersonal, systems and energy fields. Parse (1987) categorised theories under the 'simultaneity' and 'totality' paradigms.

Perhaps one of the most enduring methods of categorising theories is to allocate them to one or more broader 'worldview' paradigms. It may at first appear confusing but all practice theories regardless of discipline may have their roots in these broader paradigms; nursing theories are no exception. The paradigms have been identified as systems, interactional and developmental (Stevens Barnum 1998). Some theories also have a large behavioural basis, and so we include the behavioural paradigm as a fourth category (Grahame 1987).

Systems paradigm

Systems paradigm theories are largely based upon the 'general systems' paradigm as put forward by Von Bertalanffy (1951). Put simply, a system is a collection of parts that function as a whole entity for a particular purpose. Therefore, the parts within a particular system are interrelated. These interrelationships may form subsystems within the parent system. Similarly, the system itself may form part of an overall suprasystem. If the system has permeable boundaries it is called an open system. In system theories, the patient is often referred to as an open system. The work of Roy (1970), Neuman (Neuman & Young 1972), Johnson (1959), Parse (1981) and Fitzpatrick (Fitzpatrick & Whall 1983) may be subsumed under the systems paradigm.

Activity 4: Systems

A system is made up of subsystems. Think of the human body as a system with subsystems being the respiratory system, cardiac system, and so on. But systems exist in a larger suprasystem (e.g. family, class grouping). This system interacts with other systems and has permeable boundaries because there are inputs into the system (knowledge, food, water, and so on) and outputs (waste, speech, perspiration, and so on).

   Think of a hospital ward as a system. What subsystems could exist in that system? What suprasystem is the ward part of and what are the inputs and outputs to the system? What are the permeable boundaries that exist between this system and other similar systems?

   Identify two other things that may be conceptualised as a system.

Interactional paradigm

Interactional theories have their origin in the symbolic interactionist paradigm (Blumer 1969). This paradigm emphasises the relationships between people and the roles they play in society. Nursing activities are perceived as interactional processes between practitioners and patients. Among the better-known interactional theories are those of Riehl (1974), Orlando (1961), Patterson and Zderad (1976), Levine (1966) and King (1968).

   Take the example of a nurse assessing a patient: an interaction is taking place where a transaction of information occurs. Furthermore, the interaction, and the results of it, may be decided by the various roles the practitioner and the patient play. The nurse also reacts to the patient's interaction and vice versa and may alter their own interactional processes as a result of reactions from the patient. Therefore, we hope you can see how the interactional theories can be applied to a practice situation.

Developmental paradigm

The developmental paradigm originated from the work of Freud (1949) and Sullivan (1953). The central themes are growth, development, maturation and change. It is argued that human beings are constantly developing, whether physiologically, socially, psychologically or spiritually. Development is seen as an ongoing process in which the person must pass through various stages. The nurse's role is to encourage positive development and to break down or discourage the formation of barriers to natural development. The works of Peplau (1952), Travelbee (1966) and Newman (1979) are often perceived as having their foundations in developmental theory.

Within a developmental paradigm, nurses often encourage growth and development much as a gardener would do with plants. The patient may have had a stroke and have to live with a new disability or be a mother who has given birth to a handicapped child. Initially, care will be required for these patients to learn new attitudes, knowledge and skills in order to mature in the new situation in which they find themselves. Hopefully, their care will reach a point where they will no longer require the support and presence of the nurse or midwife because they will have changed to a higher level of growth within the limits of the disabilities.

Behavioural paradigm

Behavioural paradigm theories owe much to the theoretical formulations of Abraham Maslow (1954). Because of this, they are often referred to as 'human needs' theories (Webb 1986). Behavioural theories assume that individuals normally exist and survive by meeting their own needs. Included in this category is the work of Henderson (Henderson & Harmer 1955), Roper et al. (1980), Orem (1958), Minshull et al. (1986) and Wiedenbach (1964).

Because there are no rigid criteria available to classify theories, disagreements have occurred among authors as to which grouping a particular theory belongs. For instance, Orem's work has been seen as having its basis in the systems paradigm by Suppe and Jacox (1985), in the interactional paradigm by Greaves (1984), in the developmental paradigm by McFarlane (1986) and in the behavioural paradigm by Chapman (1985). Notwithstanding these disagreements, this method of classification has been considered a valid one for categorising nursing theories.

The metaparadigm

In other parts of this book we refer to the metaparadigm. Here we will provide a fuller account of it. Regardless of how theories are categorised, there is a consensus of opinion that each one must specify certain central concepts. These have been identified as nursing, health, the person and the environment (Yura & Torres 1975). These 'essential elements' of a theory have been referred to as the 'metaparadigm' of nursing (Fawcett 2005).

Fawcett pointed out that every discipline singles out certain phenomena with which it will uniquely deal and such phenomena coalesce to form the metaparadigm for that discipline. She described a metaparadigm as the most global perspective of a discipline acting as an encapsulating unit or framework within which the more restricted structures develop. For example, the metaparadigm used by architects or aerospace engineers would be considerably different to that used by nurses. Most professions have a single metaparadigm from which numerous theories emerge – contemporary nursing appears to have reached this level of theoretical sophistication.

During the 1970s and 1980s authors wrote extensively about the importance of these essential elements for nursing science. The argument was put forward that if a nursing theory did not include assumptions about nursing, health, person and environment it could not be considered to be a theory.

Activity 5: The metaparadigm

With three or four of your colleagues spend 15 minutes considering what you think 'nursing', 'health', 'person' and 'environment' mean to each of you. Write one sentence on each and try and refrain from using quotations from well-known theorists. Once this is complete, compare your ideas with what your colleagues have written, and then as a group attempt to categorise your views within the four paradigms: the systems, interactional, developmental or behavioural paradigm.

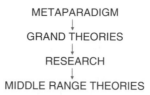

METAPARADIGM
↓
GRAND THEORIES
↓
RESEARCH
↓
MIDDLE RANGE THEORIES

Figure 5.3 The influence of the metaparadigm on the development of grand and middle range theories.

The complete four-element metaparadigm has its dissenters. For example, Stevens Barnum (1998) excluded environment, while Kim (1983) excluded health. Others believe that nursing should be omitted as a concept, maintaining that its inclusion is a redundancy in terms and that caring should be included (Leininger cited in Huch 1995). Nonetheless, the retention of metaparadigmatic intactness has been strongly supported by Fawcett (2005).

Since the metaparadigm represents the foundation stones for various theories, one would expect each theory to outline its beliefs and assumptions regarding the person, to present an identification of the person's environment, to define its conceptualisation of nursing (and/or midwifery) and to discuss the theorist's views on health.

Although each grand theory conceptualises the four essential elements of the metaparadigm, they tend to view them from different perspectives (Figure 5.3). Therefore, how nursing, health, person and environment are described and defined varies greatly from theorist to theorist. Thus, while authors consider the same metaparadigm they may emphasise different aspects and see them in different relations to one another. Such a rich diversity of assumptions concerning the same factors will only serve to enrich our profession.

Below we have extracted the metaparadigm components from the works of Henderson (1966), Roper et al. (1980), Orem (1980) and Roy (1971). See which ones you favour.

Person

'Biological human beings with inseparable mind and body who share certain fundamental human needs.' (Henderson 1966)

'An unfragmented whole who carries out or is assisted in carrying out those activities that contribute to the process of living.' (Roper et al. 1980)

'A functional integrated whole with a motivation to achieve self care.' (Orem 1980)

'A biopsychosocial being who presents as an integrated whole.' (Roy 1971)

Nursing

'A profession that assists the person sick or well in the performance of those activities contributing to health or its recovery (or to a peaceful death) that he would perform unaided if he had the necessary strength, will, or knowledge.' (Henderson 1966)

'A profession whose focus is to help the patient to prevent, solve, alleviate, or cope with problems associated with the activities he carries out in order to live.' (Roper et al. 1980)

'A human service related to the patients' need and ability to undertake self care and to help them sustain health, recover from disease and injury or cope with their effects.' (Orem 1980)

'A socially valued service whose goal is to promote a positive adaptation to the stimuli and stresses encountered by the patient.' (Roy 1971)

Health

'The ability to function independently regarding fourteen activities of daily living.' (Henderson 1966)

'The optimum level of independence in each activity of living which enables the individual to function at his/her maximum potential.' (Roper et al. 1980)

'A state of wholeness or integrity of the individual, his parts and his modes of functioning.' (Orem 1980)

'The adaptation of the person to stimuli on a continuous line between wellness and illness.' (Roy 1971)

Environment

'That which may act in a positive or negative way upon the patient.' (Henderson 1966)

'Circumstances that may impinge upon the person as he travels along the lifespan and cause movement towards maximum dependence or maximum independence.' (Roper et al. 1980)

'A subcomponent of man, and with man forms an integrated system related to self care.' (Orem 1980)

'Both internal and external. From the environment man is subject to stresses.' (Roy 1971)

Limitations of nursing theories

Grand theories used in nursing have not gone without criticism, nor have their disadvantages been ignored (summarised in Table 5.2). Two major denunciations have already been alluded to in previous chapters, namely, the belief that most are abstract non-testable conceptual models (Fawcett 1995), and that there are so many theories that it is difficult for practitioners to be familiar with them all (Clark 1986).

Webb (1986) differentiates between low-level and high-level criticisms, the former being more easily overcome than the latter.

Low-level criticisms

Documentation

The emphasis on increased paperwork when using theories has alienated many practitioners. For most nurses the implementation of theories is seen as a 'paper' exercise. For example, according to Miller (1985), Roy's theory required 16 A4 pages for its proper application!

The suitability of American theories

As outlined above, most nursing theories have their origin in the USA. A question has been posed as to whether these theories are transferable to practice in Britain. Wright (1986) suggested that there is nothing wrong with professionals from different nations swapping ideas, but the application of one group's practices to the other may not always be appropriate. Therefore, if British nurses continually look towards America for conceptual guidance, a manipulative process will have to be employed to assure the validity of US theories within the National Health Service. You must also be aware that nursing theories from the USA have their roots in a different culture, a different healthcare structure and a different training scheme.

Jargon

Most of the available theories are characterised by elaborate abstruse language. This has been referred to as 'abstract jargon' (Wright 1985), 'verbal diarrhoea' (Houlihan 1986) and 'semantic confusion' (Hardy

1986). This contributes much to the unmanageability of theories in practice. There is also the danger that the use of this 'jargonese' will lead to widespread confusion not only among practising nurses but also among the public and our multidisciplinary colleagues.

In a later chapter we will discuss the term 'parsimony'. Suffice to say here that parsimony dictates that all theories should be elegant in their simplicity (Walker & Avant 1995). In other words a good theory is stated in the simplest terms possible. Therefore, the theorist has a responsibility to put forward their theory in as simple a form as possible.

Unfortunately, most nursing theories have paid little attention to the concept of parsimony. For example, Rogers (1970) is quoted as emphasising the need to avoid jargon, yet she sees the environment as 'a four-dimensional negatrophic energy field identified by pattern and organisation, and encompassing all that is outside any given human field'. The language usage within other theories is just as perplexing and may lead to confusion. For example, 'adaptation' in one theory (Roy 1971) is taken to mean something totally different from 'adaptation' in another theory (Levine 1966). Similarly a 'stressor' is viewed as a negative stimulus in one theory (Roy 1971), while it is defined as a positive force in another (Neuman & Young 1972).

Although acknowledging the overuse of jargon in theories, Aggleton and Chalmers (2000) believed its identification as a major criticism was unduly cynical. Theory must have complexity to be significant. After all, since the concepts under study are abstract, precise theoretical language must, by necessity, be complex. The problem is not only unique to theories within our discipline: remember that Freud's theory introduced the terms ego, superego, id, Oedipus complex, Electra complex, and so on.

Webb (1986) believed that practitioners have a professional obligation to make an effort to understand the vernacular of theories. After all, she pointed out, the learning of any new subject, be it music, law, or gardening, requires that the student becomes familiar with a new language.

Staffing issues

There is much discussion in the national press about nursing shortages. If a theory identifies goals that cannot be met due to lack of time, the hard-pressed nurse is likely to become extremely frustrated. This may also raise ethical issues. One wonders if it is morally right to uncover multiple problems with a patient when, because of staff shortages or short lengths of stay, only a few will be addressed. There is also the argument that in a ward where individualised patient care is practised, there will be different staffing requirements than in a ward that practises the 'block treatment' method of task-oriented care.

High-level criticisms

Conceptual substance

Many theories have been criticised for adopting a restricting view of nursing. Some authors believe that theorists have trodden a narrow path in their efforts to theorise. The medical model has been castigated for its emphasis on reductionism. However, as alluded to elsewhere in this book, the theories of Roper, Roy, Henderson, King and Orem *reduce* the patient to a list of activities, needs, modes of adapting or to a set of self-care needs.

There is also the contrary accusation that in an attempt to be all-inclusive, nursing theories provide inadequate guidance for practice. The belief that these broad grand theories are general statements about care has led some to the idea that a theory can be utilised in a wide range of settings. This blanket application of one theory may, according to Hardy (1986), be unwise and even dangerous.

Ideal concepts vs practical reality

Most theories deal with practice as it ought to be, and not as it is. However, if we do not know what nursing or midwifery is, how can we work within the real world of practice? Meleis (2007), in considering this problem, felt that theorists were becoming more competent in articulating what theory is, rather than what is the substance of practice itself.

Nurses are often characterised as being anti-intellectual when it comes to research and theories. Although the apparent gap between what theorists believe and what goes on in the busy clinical setting is one reason for this, the imposition of theories by management encourages such reactions. The introduction by force of a theory that is supposed to be based upon individual choice is an obvious contradiction.

Therefore, those who wish to introduce a theory into the clinical setting may be met by sceptical practitioners who see theories as merely the results of academic exercises aimed at increasing the complexities of their working lives. Within the UK, nursing theories have taken over the unpopular position previously occupied by the nursing process.

Benefits of nursing theories

Those who advocate the use of theories do so for a number of reasons, summarised in Table 5.1. Two distinct benefits have already been discussed. These are, the substitution of nursing theories for the medical model for delivering care, and the understanding that theories lead to the development of nursing knowledge. These are without doubt important gains both for patients and professionals. However, the literature highlights several other equally favourable advantages.

A guide for practice

There is consensus of opinion for the suggestion that the implementation of the nursing process without a theory to underpin it is an empty approach often described as 'practising in the dark' (Aggleton & Chalmers 2000). Although British nurses have only been recently introduced to theories, they have been wrestling with the nursing process for some time. It could be argued that they have got the 'cart before the horse'. By providing a systematic basis for assessment, planning, implementing and evaluating, theories offer a way to revitalise the nursing process.

Therefore, in order to be implemented successfully and to have meaning for practitioners, the nursing process as a problem-solving exercise must be framed within a theory. As a supplement to this role, nursing theories also stress the importance of the wholeness and integrity of the person, thus further enhancing the practitioner's ability to provide individualised care. These theories are essential guides for practice, and as such they help bring theory and practice closer together.

The usefulness of these frameworks has also been recognised in the areas of nursing education, administration and research (Nicholl 1992).

Education

Although the dichotomy between classroom and ward is well documented (Meleis 2007), evidence exists to suggest that the structuring of an education programme around a theory is extremely beneficial for students (Aggleton & Chalmers 2000) and, as a result, theory and practice may eventually meet.

Professionalisation

The use of theory as a basis for practice is one of the characteristics of a profession. Smith (1986) maintained that nursing could achieve full professional status comparable with other professions by basing its practice on theories. Theories were also seen as harbingers of autonomy and responsibility, leading to professional accountability (Meleis 2007).

Quality of care

In his research, McKenna (1994) found that the quality of care given by a practitioner using a theory is high because practice is built on a systematic knowledge base. There is a strong indication that nurses must practise from a theoretical foundation if care is to be of good quality.

The quality of a service cannot be assessed unless there are standards against which an appraisal can be made. Quality of care evaluation in contemporary practice is becoming increasingly related to cost effectiveness. If used appropriately, nursing theories can demonstrate cost effectiveness through reducing dependency, encouraging self-care, and the early detection of patients' problems. In addition, a theory also allows staff a greater articulation of health goals, hence identifying more efficiently the resources and skills needed to achieve them.

Tables 5.1 and 5.2 summarise the major benefits and limitations of theories for practice. These statements have been obtained from the literature. However, be aware that most are opinions rather than evidenced through research – so some are contradictory:

Table 5.1 Perceived benefits of theories for practice.

Assists student learning
Helps to structure patient assessment
Permits meaningful communication between nurses
Improves problem-solving
Increases patients' satisfaction
Identifies the goals of practice
Substantially improves quality of care
Clarifies nurses' realm of accountability
Focuses observations on important phenomena
Guides and justifies actions
Clarifies thinking among nurses about practice
Provides others with a rationale for nurses' work
Directs research into clinical needs

Table 5.2 Perceived limitations of models for practice.

Does not prepare nurses for the reality of practice
Offers little guidance for action
Too abstract, academic, idealistic and irrelevant
Is not responsible for any change in practice
Leads to premature closure on ideas
Its application is a criticism of current practice
Provides only the illusion of positive change
Misleads practitioners because they are not reality
Provides only tentative ideas about practice
Unable to cope with multiple clinical foci
Not empirically tested or evaluated in practice

Summary

In the 1950s in the USA a group of nurses began to theorise about practice. Thirty years later, nurses in the UK began to study and use some of these theories and some others formulated British theories. Most of these theories can trace their origin to one of four influential paradigms: systems, interactional, behavioural and developmental. Furthermore, each theory has something to say about the essential elements of the metaparadigm.

On both sides of the Atlantic nursing theories have been lauded by some and criticised by others. Much time has been spent discussing whether they are theories at all. A body of opinion argued that most are better referred to as models. The point of view adopted in this book is to leave behind the debate on semantics, accept that there are theories at different stages of development and concentrate on the use and testing of these theories in practice.

Nursing Theories and Interpersonal Relationships

'No man is an island, entire of itself; every man is a piece of the continent, a part of the main; if a clod be washed away by the sea, Europe is the less; as well as if a promontory were, as well as if a manor of thy friends or of thine own were; any man's death diminishes me, because I am involved in mankind . . .'

Meditation XVII, John Donne (1571–1631)

Outline of content

This chapter consists of three interrelated parts. First of all it explores the centrality of interpersonal relations for the profession and discipline of nursing. Second, it outlines a number of nursing theories that have interpersonal relations at their core. You will not be surprised that most of this focuses on the work of Hildegard Peplau. Finally, ideas are presented about how best to educate nurses to develop and sustain positive interpersonal relationships with patients, families and communities and the potential barriers to achieving these goals.

John Donne's famous words illustrate that being human is about connecting with other human beings. Readers will be aware of the psychological experiments that have taken place where subjects were placed in an isolation chamber for long periods of time. The negative effects are well documented: the psychological effects of isolation include anxiety, depression, sleep disturbance, withdrawal, regression and hallucinations.

But there are different types of isolation. Nurses often encounter people who are isolated within their own communities. For instance, Lane and co-workers carried out a study on the experiences of home-based carers looking after family members who had dementia. They found that many carers referred to the sense of isolation they experienced and the difficulties they encountered that were associated with not being able to maintain normal social and interpersonal relationships with anyone other than the demented person being cared for (Lane et al. 2003).

However, interpersonal relationships are only one dimension of human functioning. Hoff (1995) suggested that a crisis such as any kind of illness will only be resolved if there are mediating factors. He identified these mediating factors as intrapersonal, interpersonal and extrapersonal. Intrapersonal factors are internal to the individual and include their perception of the crisis, past experiences of the disease and the individuals' emotional and physical health. Interpersonal mediating factors include family networks, professional input and social support. Extrapersonal factors include timing and duration of the crisis, financial resources and competing family and work obligations. The emphasis within this chapter will be on interpersonal factors.

The term 'interpersonal relations' was first coined in 1941 by Jacob Moreno, a psychiatrist who founded psychodrama. It was later defined more precisely by the psychoanalyst Harry Stack Sullivan (1953). It forms the basis for all human connections whether this is with family, friends, neighbours, work colleagues, or simply other members of the community with whom we interact fleetingly.

As nurses the authors often witnessed how poor and unstable interpersonal relationships led to mental health problems and also how the development of stable interpersonal relationships brought people back to good mental health. It can be argued that most mental illnesses stem from interpersonal relationship problems. But such relationships are not just important for mental health nursing. They are core elements of the caring repertoires of all nurses in every field.

In research with patients who had a diagnosis of cancer, McCaughan and McKenna (2007) noted that good-quality care occurred in a very specific interpersonal atmosphere. Patients were clear that they gained a sense of relief by being able to talk about their feelings, thoughts and experiences within a therapeutic relationship. In such a relationship they felt that they were allowed the freedom to express themselves and as a result they had a feeling of security and a sense of emancipation. Interestingly though, there was something qualitatively different about the patients' relationship with the nurse as opposed to their relationship with their family and friends. In the latter relationships, feelings were expressed sparingly for fear of causing pain or distress whereas feelings and fears were expressed freely to nurses. This supports Peplau's assertion that the relationship between nurse and patient is not the same as the more common social relationships:

> 'The nurse patient relationship is a particular kind of interaction. It is not a social relationship of friend to friend. It is not a clerk to customer relationship. Nor is it a master to servant relationship. Rather, the nurse is a professional, which means a person having a definable expertise. That expertise pertains to reliable interventions which have been research tested and therefore have predictable known outcomes.' (Peplau 1992: 14)

Therefore the interpersonal relationships between patients and nurses form a core element within the caring process. Caring has always been and will always be about humans interacting with humans in a mutually respectful partnership. The essence of these partnerships is the facilitation of the growth and development of therapeutic relationships. Support for this can be found in Canadian research undertaken by Janice Morse (1995). She identified five types of caring:

- caring as an affect
- caring as a human trait
- caring as a moral imperative
- caring as a therapeutic intervention
- caring as an interpersonal relationship.

She stressed that building and sustaining interpersonal relationships are pivotal to caring. More recently, Fosbinder (1994) showed that the quality of care received by patients was related to the quality of the interpersonal relationships they had with nurses. Patients value interpersonal relationships very highly and this is often what leads to high patient satisfaction.

A note of caution though; when we discuss interpersonal relationships we often think of the positive and life-enhancing aspects, but of course there can be relationships between persons that are negative and damaging. Theoretically, positive interpersonal relationships are composed of concepts such as trust, hope, understanding, empathy, respect and admiration, to name just a few. In contrast, negative interpersonal relationships are reflected in concepts such as distrust, anger, disrespect, disapproval and dislike. The role of the nurse is to encourage the formation of positive interpersonal relationships and eliminate or discourage the formation of those that are negative. Many nursing theories act as guides to show how best to do this.

Activity 1: What is caring?

Many people and organisations pride themselves on being caring. The pilots who fly you off on holiday see their role as caring, as do shop assistants, police officers, doctors and firefighters.

Using your library resources, look up caring in nursing. You may wish to consult some nursing theories that have caring as their focus such as those of Madeleine Leininger or Jean Watson.

Once you have read some work on caring, write a page on why you believe nurses are caring and whether you believe they are different in their caring to those in the occupations outlined above.

Interpersonal theories of nursing

From Chapter 3 you will remember that Carper wrote on knowing in nursing (Carper 1978). Based on earlier work in 1975, she identified four types of knowing: *empirics*, the science of nursing (including theories); *aesthetics*, the art of nursing; *ethics*, moral knowing; and *personal knowing*. We are surprised that there was not an interpersonal way of knowing. We suspect Carper would argue that it is inherent in all four ways of knowing or embedded within her 'personal knowing' category.

According to Carper, 'personal knowing' is subjective; it is about nurses knowing themselves and how they relate to others. It represents knowledge that focuses on self-consciousness, personal awareness and empathy. It requires self-regard, and active empathic participation on the part of the nurse. Why is personal knowing so important in the context of this chapter? Well, if we accept that nursing is an interpersonal process then we must know our own strengths and weaknesses in order to be able to interact meaningfully with those requiring our care. After all, most nurses do not possess a case full of medications or an arsenal of surgical instruments: what we have is ourselves and we can use ourselves therapeutically to make a difference to patients. This requirement to know ourselves before we can know our patients forms part of several nursing theories.

As alluded to previously, research by McKenna (1994) noted that there were over 50 nursing theories. He studied each of these in some depth and found that to a greater or lesser extent all of them refer to interaction between nurses and patients. This will not surprise you since a nursing theory that does not refer to such interactions would not be worthy of the title 'nursing theory'. Nonetheless, some theories place a greater emphasis on interpersonal processes than others.

However, before we explore this further, it might be useful to remind you once again what a theory is:

> 'A set of concepts, definitions and propositions that project a systematic view of phenomena by designating specific interrelationships among concepts for the purpose of describing, explaining, predicting and/or controlling phenomena.' (Chinn & Kramer 2004)

In her textbook, Afaf Meleis (1985, 1991, 1997, 2007) noted that there were three categories of nursing theories: needs theories, outcome theories and interaction theories.

Theories in the first category focus on answering the question *What do nurses do?* These tend to centre on providing assistance with activities of living as outlined by Virginia Henderson (1966), or self-care needs as outlined by Dorothea Orem (1980). What nurses do is also reflected in those theories that centre on general human needs such as the work of Jean Minshull (Minshull et al. 1986) or Faye Abdellah (Abdellah et al. 1960). These theories are also closely tied to the medical model (referred to in Chapter 4) because, if you examine them closely, you will see that physical needs and medical needs have a prominent position within them.

Theories in the second category focus on answering the question *Why is nursing needed?* These tended to concentrate on the outcomes of the caring process and include the work of Dorothy Johnson (1959), Martha Rogers (1970) and Callista Roy (1971).

The third groups of theories are the ones that we are particularly interested in for this chapter. They seek to answer the question *How do nurses do whatever it is they do?* These are referred to as interaction theories. They were conceived in the 1950s and early 1960s and the most renowned are those of Hildegard Peplau (1952), Ida Orlando (1961), Joyce Travelbee (1966) and Imogene King (1968). In the parlance used by us in previous chapters these are grand theories rather than middle range or practice theories.

This group of theorists tended to view nursing as an interactional process that is concerned with the development of a therapeutic interpersonal relationship between patients and nurses. Four tables show how similar or different these theories are with regard to their definitions (Table 6.1), focus (Table 6.2), goals (Table 6.3) and interventions (Table 6.4). They are based on an analysis carried out by Meleis (2007).

Peplau (1988) defined nursing as a therapeutic interpersonal process while Travelbee (1966) asserted that nursing is an interpersonal process between two human beings, one of who needs assistance because of an illness and the other who is able to give such assistance. Orlando (1961) emphasised that the nurse–patient relationship should be based on

Table 6.1 How interpersonal theories define nursing.

Theorist	Definition of nursing
Peplau 1952	A therapeutic interpersonal goal-oriented process: a health-focused human relationship
Orlando 1961	Interaction with patients who have a need or response to individuals who are suffering
Travelbee 1966	An interpersonal process to prevent or cope with experiences of illness and find meaning in this
King 1968	Action, reaction and interaction where the nurse and patient share information and agree on goals

Table 6.2 How interpersonal theories denote the focus of nursing.

Theorist	Focus of nursing
Peplau 1952	Phases of nurse–patient relationship – orientation, identification, exploitation and resolution
Orlando 1961	Care of the needs of patients who are distressed through deliberate action
Travelbee 1966	Interpersonal relations – finding meaning in suffering, pain and illness
King 1968	Nurse–patient interactions that lead to goal attainment in a natural environment

Table 6.3 How interpersonal theories denote the goals of nursing.

Theorist	Goals of nursing
Peplau 1952	Develop personality in creative, constructive, productive personal and community living
Orlando 1961	Relieve distress, physical and mental discomfort and promote a sense of wellbeing
Travelbee 1966	Cope with an illness situation and find meaning in the experience
King 1968	Help individuals maintain their health so that they can function in their role

Table 6.4 How interpersonal theories denote nursing interventions.

Theorist	Nursing interventions
Peplau 1952	Develop problem-solving skills in patients through therapeutic interpersonal processes
Orlando 1961	Deliberate nursing process, where nurse uses interpersonal skills to address patient's distress
Travelbee 1966	Use of nurse's self and empathy, support and rapport to understand the patient's pain
King 1968	Goal attainment, transaction and perceptual validation as part of the nurse–patient interaction

planned action. King's theory (1968) focused on nursing as a process of human interaction between the nurse and patient, whereby each perceives the other in the situation and through communication they set goals, and explore and agree on the means to achieve goals.

These theorists have their basis in a mixture of existential philosophy, symbolic interactionism and developmental theory. They provide four lessons for nurses (after Meleis 2007):

1 Nursing is an interpersonal process occurring between a person in need of help and a person capable of giving help.
2 To be able to give help, the nurse should clarify and understand her own values (Carper's personal knowing; 1978): without this she will not be able to establish connections with patients and give care in a therapeutic way.
3 Nurse–patient relationships are formed to relieve distress as well as to enhance trust.
4 The patient is an equal partner in the care process and the perceptions of patients are important in assessing illness and its meaning.

Table 6.4 outlines the interventions recommended by these theorists.

Activity 2: Which is your preferred theory?

Read the above descriptions of the four theories and decide what one best fits with your perspective on interpersonal relationships. If you require more information before you make up your mind, please refer to other articles and books by the theorists.

Continued

> Write a short piece on why you made your choice. Compare this with other students to see if they have selected the same theory as you have. If not, what reasons could there be for the difference?

Space does not permit us to discuss the four theories in detail. However, we will select Peplau's as she can rightly be regarded as the mother of interaction theories. Hers was the first contemporary theory in nursing generally and psychiatric nursing in particular. Her writings in the 1950s greatly influenced others who later used interpersonal relationships as a basis for their theories.

From her long and distinguished experience as a psychiatric nurse, Peplau realised that people who have good mental health often have good interpersonal relationships with others such as their family, friends and work colleagues. Conversely, she noted that people who were psychiatrically unwell invariably had poor interpersonal skills and had difficulty communicating appropriately with others. You recall in Chapter 3 we discussed how knowledge can be built through induction, deduction or retroduction. Hildegard Peplau studied interpersonal relations over many years and began to develop her theory deductively through the influence of Harry Stack Sullivan's (1953) interpersonal relations theory and inductively through reflecting on her clinical experience in psychiatric nursing. Interestingly, Peplau never actually used the term 'interpersonal relationships', preferring instead to use 'interpersonal relations'. This may be due simply to her respect for Harry Stack Sullivan's theory.

Peplau (1952) defined nursing as a therapeutic interpersonal process through which nurses facilitate growth and development among patients. She saw the relationship as reciprocal with both the nurse and the patient participating in and contributing to it.

You will note from a previous chapter that theories often have a number of assumptions. These are simply statements that we accept as true even though they may not have been proved. The following example from Callista Roy's theory illustrates what an assumption is. Among other assumptions, she stated that all people have biopsychosocial dimensions and that they constantly adapt to a changing environment.

Consider the following assumptions from Peplau and reflect if they are still relevant for nursing in the 21st century:

'People need relationships with other people.' (Peplau 1995b: 67)

'Relationships constitute the social fabric of life.' (Peplau 1995b: 66)

'Interpersonal relationships are important throughout the life-span.' (Peplau 1992: 34)

'Interpersonal relationships are the bedrock of quality of life.' (Peplau 1992: 33)

'In every nurse–patient contact there is the possibility of working towards common understandings and goals.' (Peplau 1952: 10)

'The nurse and patient come to know and to respect each other as persons who are alike and yet different, as persons who share in the solution of problems.' (Peplau 1952: 9)

'Each patient–nurse relationship is unique in terms of process and outcome.' (Peplau 1962: 5)

'Interpersonal relationships are person-to-person interactions that have structure and content and are situation dependent.' (Peplau 1992: 34)

'At their best, interpersonal relationships confirm self worth, provide a sense of connectedness with others and support self esteem.' (Peplau 1995b: 66)

We are sure no sensible reader would disagree with any of these statements and recognise their pertinence for nursing today and in the future. Let's have a closer look at her theory (Table 6.5).

To Peplau, the interpersonal process has a starting point called the 'orientation phase' when the nurse and patient are strangers to each other; it proceeds through the 'working phase' and, being time limited, has an end point at the 'termination phase'. Across these phases Peplau (1988) proposed that the nurse's role changes as she interacts with patients. From the table, readers can see that the various roles are 'counsellor', 'resource person', 'leader', 'teacher' and 'surrogate sibling'. By adopting these roles, nurses rely more on guiding, supporting, teaching and helping patients to find meaning in their situations – and less on doing and functioning.

Table 6.5 Phases and roles within Peplau's theory.

Phases in relationship	Orientation phase		Working phase	Terminal phase
Patient's role	stranger	infant/child	adolescent	adult person
Nurse's role	stranger	unconditional, mother surrogate	counsellor, resource person, leader, teacher, surrogate sibling	adult person

> **Activity 3: Peplau's theory**
>
> Look at Table 6.5 above. A nurse might be a resource person if the patient or patient's family wanted health promotion information or literature. She might adopt the role of teacher if she was showing a diabetic patient how to administer insulin.
>
> Identify three situations when a nurse would adopt each of the roles in the working phase of the theory.

Unfortunately, there remains a dearth of research into the empirical testing of the interaction theories. This reflects the situation with most nursing theories. We believe more investigations are needed to discover the ways in which these relationships are nurtured, supported, discouraged or avoided. Some of these answers may be found in the philosophical, sociology and social psychology literature but we must also generate our own body of empirical evidence in this area. We would reiterate the call for a moratorium on theory development until some of the ones that already exist have been tested and evaluated.

Implications for nurse education

Considering their centrality to nursing you would expect that there should be a strong emphasis on interpersonal relationships in nurse education curricula and that interpersonal theories should be used as a framework to structure such curricula. From existing evidence, this is not the case.

The reasons are obvious: general nursing curricula are packed with everything from anatomy and physiology to practical tasks and research methods. The examination of interpersonal relationships constitutes a small part of such programmes. Also, nursing theories no longer have the popularity they had in the 1980s; back then it was not possible to pick up a journal or a textbook without seeing them mentioned. Today they are mostly absent from curricula and journal articles.

There is an opportunity for nurse educators to redress this void and develop an interpersonal culture of education. Within such a culture nurses could learn the following:

- To acknowledge that interpersonal relationships are the foundation stone of quality care.
- To see themselves and the particular ways in which they talk to each other and to patients as part of the therapeutic process.

- To accept interpersonal responsibility and encourage open, sensitive personal relations and strong feelings of interpersonal trust.
- To develop their personal knowing so that they have a good understanding of their own values, attitudes and knowledge for this will determine the extent to which the nurse can understand the situation confronting the patient.
- To observe and record their own behaviour in the classroom and get detailed feedback from their fellow students and from teachers in order to understand the impact of their own words, actions and reactions on each other and on their learning.
- To be sensitive to the human problems that confront patients and be able to develop with patients the kind of relationship that will be conducive to dealing with these problems.

Social capital

Another way of viewing interpersonal relationships is through the phenomenon called social capital. There are three kinds of capital – economic capital, human capital and social capital. The most important type of capital in this context is social capital, a term first used in 1972 by Pierre Bourdieu (Bourdieu 1977). One way to understand this concept is to take the two words that comprise social capital: social, meaning relating to humans, and capital, meaning wealth. Within the context of interpersonal relationships, nurses must be educated to become expert in developing this social wealth in themselves and in patients.

According to Cohen and Prusak:

> 'Social capital consists of the stock of active connections among people: the trust, mutual understanding, and shared values and behaviors that bind the members of human networks and communities and make cooperative action possible.' (Cohen & Prusak 2001: 4)

Therefore, social capital is the values and norms that individuals share with others that permit relationship building.

This ability to generate social capital within nursing not only benefits patients directly but also multidisciplinary team working. It is a truism that modern healthcare is mainly provided through multiprofessional team members bringing their own skills and competencies to the clinical situation. Skills in interpersonal relationships are crucial for effective teamworking. As alluded to elsewhere in this book, if different members of the multidisciplinary team have the same theoretical leanings, it makes the team stronger and more cohesive and is less confusing for patients.

When Charlton was speaking about multidisciplinary working over 25 years ago he used the following analogy:

'We are like inhabitants of a number of little islands all in the same part of the ocean. Each has evolved a different culture, different ways of doing things and different language to talk about what they do. Occasionally the inhabitants of one island may spot their neighbours jumping up and down and issuing strange cries about some new discovery but it makes no sense to them so they ignore it.' (Charlton 1980: 15)

Such lack of team cohesion not only damages interpersonal relationships between professional colleagues but also between them and patients. One way of addressing this is to encourage interprofessional learning where different healthcare disciplines are educated together from the beginning. It teaches them that no one professional grouping owns the patient or the patient's problems. As nursing education moves increasingly into universities the opportunities for interprofessional learning will increase.

The educational challenge is to endow students with the ability to work individually or in a team, to be creative and imaginative in solving problems, to communicate clearly and effectively and to become expert in the development of interpersonal relationships. Many of these competencies are not taught in class but can be encouraged or discouraged by the pervading ethos of the university or college.

Threats to interpersonal theories and practice

Pace of modern healthcare

Many readers may remember a time when healthcare delivery was a much more relaxed endeavour. Patients often spent weeks in hospital and, as they improved, some assisted nurses to distribute meals, feed other patients and make beds. Nurses had time to get to know their patients and their patients' families.

However, in the 21st century, nursing has become 'intensified'. The fact is that now there is less time to 'nurse' than there was previously. Patient throughput has increased and new treatments and technologies have made healthcare more complex. Hospitals are little more than large intensive care units where, as soon as patients are over the acute stage of their illness, they are discharged to community care. This means that nurses have less time to get to know patients and their families. This has implications for the theories that nurses are taught and we have to ask ourselves whether detailed interpersonal theories are still relevant today.

Measuring interpersonal relationships

Healthcare managers and policy-makers are fixated on measurement. They have the adage that if it cannot be measured it cannot be costed. Most nurses are not good at explaining what they do, nor at providing evidence of effectiveness. For instance, a health service manager who sees a nurse talking to a patient in a busy clinical setting may perceive this as an example of inefficiency. The nurse may be establishing a therapeutic interpersonal relationship with the patient. However, to the untrained eye what the nurse is doing is simply talking with the patient and, after all, untrained staff can do this simple task. Interpersonal relationships are difficult to measure and thus are not easily subjected to rigorous studies of effectiveness. But we should again take comfort from Peplau, who stated:

> 'Despite our current emphasis on medical diagnoses, sophisticated technology, economic cutbacks and "quick fixes", what patients need most in the midst of this health care maze is sensitive and caring individuals who are willing to enter into interpersonal relationships that foster hope and prevent hopelessness.'
> Peplau (1995b: 67)

Increased technology

Many people commence a career in nursing because they want to help people in direct and tangible ways. Traditionally, nursing is perceived as a high 'touch' profession that values personal interaction. The need to reach out and touch someone else is just as strong in the development of interpersonal relationships with patients. Here nurses pay attention to facial expressions, body language, tone of voice and effect. This is important but presents significant challenges to education when there is a greater emphasis on e-learning and distance learning.

Increasingly, we are using technological gateways that are taking the place of face-to-face teaching. Nurses who value human contact can quite easily become frustrated simply because they are geographically removed and unable to physically connect with the person who is teaching them or their fellow students. The same can apply in clinical situations. In 1960 Isobel Menzies claimed that nurses were engaging in low-level non-nursing tasks as a defence mechanism to distance them from the stress of dealing directly with patients' problems (Menzies 1960). Peplau (1962) called this 'busywork' that kept the nurse away from direct contact with the patient. We believe that today there is still busywork to distract nurses but now it takes the form of computer technology and administrative paperwork. While the distractions have altered, they can still keep the nurse away from direct contact with patients. Nurse educators must ensure that new graduates are not enticed towards technologies as a means of isolating them physically from patients or emotionally from their patients' problems.

Role drift

In a climate of a global shortage of registered nurses and demands for them to undertake more medical duties, there is an increasing reliance on assistants to fill the gaps in care. As a result, duties and workload are shifting from doctors to nurses and from nurses to healthcare assistants. The majority of healthcare assistants are caring and conscientious individuals who are often pressurised to go beyond their level of competence to perform duties for which they are not qualified – potentially endangering patients.

Some of the duties undertaken by healthcare assistants that were once the remit of nurses include catheter care, wound dressing, venepuncture, formulating patient care plans, setting up and monitoring diagnostic machines, setting up infusion feeds, giving injections, taking charge of shifts, monitoring, providing advice on parenting skills and breast feeding. According to the literature, much of this work is unsupervised. Therefore, while many nursing roles are becoming medicalised, healthcare assistants, because of their increasing numbers and their visibility in the clinical setting, are involved more in developing interpersonal relationships with patients and their families.

We wonder if it is time to re-humanise nursing and ensure that nurses are in the best position clinically and strategically to develop therapeutic relationships with patients' families and communities. A range of well-tested nursing theories is available to help us to do so.

Summary

The focus of this chapter was on the importance of interpersonal relationships for nursing and how different theories deal with this issue. From this chapter we can be certain about six things:

1   Life generally is about interpersonal relationships.
2   Interpersonal relationships are at the core of nursing.
3   The development of positive interpersonal relationships can be therapeutic.
4   There are nursing theories that guide the development of therapeutic interpersonal relationships.
5   Nurse education has a central role to play in ensuring that nurses have the knowledge and skills necessary to develop interpersonal relationships with others.
6   There exist a number of threats to nursing's centrality in interpersonal relationships with patients. These include the pace of modern healthcare, increased technology, the inability to measure interpersonal relationships and the increased role of the healthcare assistant.

Selecting a Suitable Theory

'It is the professional practitioner who is able to criticise the theory and determine its value for directing actions to achieve defined outcomes. In this she is not only a user of theory but a modifier . . . and chooser of theory.'

Ellis (1969: 1435)

Outline of content

In this chapter it is argued that choosing an inappropriate theory for practice can have damaging effects on patient care. Conversely, a theory that is appropriate for practice will benefit patients and improve the working practices and morale of nurses. Twelve different criteria are discussed that can be used to help select a nursing theory. A number of strategies are identified to enable selection through matching your views of nursing with those of established theorists.

In the 1980s and 1990s practising nurses in the UK were to a large extent forced to use nursing theories in practice. There were a variety of reasons for this. The main reason was that such frameworks were a new fad. It was not possible to peruse a journal or attend a conference without reading or hearing about nursing theories. Invariably, clinical areas were perceived as not being up to date unless the nurses were using a nursing theory to guide practice. A second reason was that care planning and the nursing process had been introduced a few years previously and they were unpopular among clinicians and not used appropriately. There was a view in the literature that nursing theories brought the nursing process to life. In fact it had been argued that the implementation of the nursing process without a theory to underpin it is an empty approach often described as 'practising in the dark' (Aggleton & Chalmers 2000). As a result, nursing theories were perceived as the saviour to care planning and they were imposed uncritically on busy practising nurses.

It was not unusual for clinical nurses to be informed by managers that they were to introduce a nursing theory to guide their practice by the following week. Furthermore, the managers often selected the theory because they had attended a conference where the theory had been presented or had heard that it was being used in a neighbouring hospital. Another common reason was that nurse teachers in the local school of nursing were teaching the specific theory to their students or it underpinned the curriculum.

When choosing a nursing theory little consideration was given to patient needs or the clinical specialty. In the UK, the theories selected most often had more than a passing resemblance to the medical model. For instance, Henderson's theory (1966) or that of Roper et al. (2000) were the most popular choices whether the patient population was people with mental health problems, women in labour, sick children, or older people. Wimpenny (2002) criticised this, highlighting the advantage in matching particular theories to particular specialties. After all, he argued, different theories had been developed from a particular experiential perspective.

Chapman (1990) related a typical UK selection strategy:

'Senior nurses and tutors decide which theory will be used in each ward or unit and charge nurses and staff are requested to become acquainted with it (with varying amounts of help from the school and service side) and to interpret and use it on their ward. Enthusiasm . . . may understandably be grudging, so the minimum is done to satisfy the requirements.' (Chapman 1990: 14).

In McKenna's study (1994) it was noted that there were over 50 grand theories of nursing and a growing number of middle range theories. Since assessment of need, planning care, interventions and evaluation of care will differ depending on what theory is being used, a new awareness exists as to the necessity of making an appropriate choice. However, there is a dearth of research available as to which theory is best suited for which specialty. For instance, in a psychiatric unit where the development of interpersonal relationships is important, would Peplau's theory (1992) be most appropriate? But the theories of Orlando

(1961), Travelbee (1966), King (1968), Wiedenbach (1964) and Patterson and Zderad (1976) also focus on interpersonal relationships. As a result, choosing the most relevant theory is a daunting task and must be carried out with care.

It could be argued that grand theories are so broad in their scope that they should be applicable in any setting where nursing is taking place. For instance, Orem's self-care theory (1980) could be used in any setting where patients are being encouraged to be independent. This would give it wide applicability. So, is sorting through theories to find a suitable one a waste of your valuable time? Stevens Barnum (1998) does not think so; she asserted that there was a need to employ different theories to suit different patient settings. We would concur with this view and argue that the choice of one theory for application throughout a hospital is imprudent. Should patients and staff have to put up with a theory that has a less desirable 'fit' for the sake of conformity to a management or educational dictat? The obvious danger is that the patient's problems would be moulded to fit the theory rather than the theory fitting patients' problems.

As stated many times in this text, grand theories are broad frameworks and often well recognised and publicised (e.g. self-care, adaptation, activities of living, and so on). In contrast, middle range theories are those that have more limited scope, less abstraction, address specific phenomena or concepts and reflect practice. Invariably, they emerge out of research studies and examples include middle range theories of uncertainty in illness (Mishel 1990), comfort (Kolcaba 2001), maternal role attainment (Mercer 1995), caring in perinatal nursing (Swanson 1991) and respite care (Nolan & Grant 1992). We would refer you back to Chapter 4 if you need to update yourself on the difference, but regardless of whether we are dealing with grand or middle range theories, we believe that there are twelve main problems in selecting an appropriate one.

Problems in selecting a theory

Ethical issues

The selection of a nursing theory is value laden and reflects Carper's (1978) 'ethical knowing'. It follows therefore that the choice will be influenced by the nurse's beliefs about and attitude to the nature of people and healthcare. For instance, Orem's self-care theory (1980) would not be a nurse's first choice if she held the view that patients are dependent and so they should adopt the sick role and do as little for themselves as possible. On the other hand, if you select a theory that encourages dependency this could do a great deal of damage to patients' rehabilitation and to their self-esteem.

More than three decades ago, Jensen (1973) fooled many US government officials with his theory that black children were less intelligent than their white counterparts. The selection of this theory to frame policy had implications for hiring employees, providing educational opportunities and the self-esteem of many people. Rigid application of the theories that the Earth was flat or that the Sun orbited around the Earth led to people like Galileo Galilei (1564–1642) being victimised and imprisoned (see Chapter 3).

Activity 1: Ethical considerations

In Chapter 5 you will recall that we discussed the barriers to the use of interactional theories to build interpersonal relationships. Among other things we mentioned the fast pace of modern healthcare and the increasing use of technology.

Also, later on in this chapter we will point out that when using a nursing theory, a nurse undertakes a comprehensive and detailed assessment and identifies many actual and potential physical, social and psychological problems. However, in the modern healthcare system the patient will only be in hospital for a short length of stay.

Write a one-page account of the ethical implications of these issues for nursing care.

Using merged or adapted theories

The idea that different concepts can be chosen from several theories and applied in the clinical area as one theory is supported by some (Fawcett 2006), but seen as totally untenable by others. Webb (1986) argued that such a strategy would lead to the loss of coherence and rigour, the introduction of contradiction, and theoretical status being compromised. More and more research is being carried out on different nursing theories and many of these studies show that a particular theory is a valid basis for guiding practice. For example, Anderson (2001) showed the effectiveness of using Orem's theory (1980) with homeless adults, and 25 years of research on Roy's theory (2003) has shown the positive outcomes of encouraging adaptation (Roy 1999). Similarly, McKenna (1994) showed that Minshull's human needs theory had a positive effect on quality of patient care. Therefore, if bits and pieces from these theories were extracted and put together to form a hybrid theory, the validity of the parent theory would be compromised and the effectiveness demonstrated by research could no longer be assured. Fawcett (2005) asserted that while modification of a theory may be acceptable, the modifications should be acknowledged and consideration should be given to renaming the theory.

Level of nurses' knowledge

While the level of knowledge about different theories will influence the selection process, readers will spot the obvious flaw with this method of selection. Considering that there are so many grand and middle range nursing theories available, is it realistic to expect busy practising nurses to be familiar with any more than a few of the most popular ones? Their level of knowledge about theories is also biased according to which theories they were taught by nurse educators and which theories achieve the highest profile in journals and books. Further bias is introduced by the type of journals the nurse reads and, as alluded to above, the predilections of nurse teachers and managers.

The growth in middle range theories complicates the selection process (see Chapter 3). It is difficult enough to have knowledge of the large number of grand theories; there are many more middle range theories (Peterson & Bredow 2004).

Social and political issues

The philosopher Paul Feyerabend (1977) argued that theory and truth cannot be divorced from the social and political context in which they exist. He maintained that the theory one chooses is a matter of social convenience or political expediency. Social and political implications also have a role to play in the selection of a nursing theory. It could be argued that Orem's work (1980) is more suitable to the private health insurance sector because of its emphasis on the patient's ability to undertake self-care as soon as possible. In modern society there is a move away from the so-called 'nanny state'. This is manifested by everything from early discharge home to the care of families, to workers being encouraged to sign up to private pensions and private health insurance. Also, the population is getting older resulting in an increase in chronic conditions and healthcare costs spiralling out of control. A self-care theory would fit well into such a world.

There is another dimension to this political influence. High-profile cases of professional misconduct such as occurred at a hospital in

Bristol and at Liverpool's Alder Hey Hospital, and serial killers Dr Harold Shipman and nurse Beverly Allitt have shaken people's confidence in health professionals. Nurses are more accountable now than at any other time and members of the public are rightly asking increasingly perceptive questions about their care and treatment. If nurses commit themselves to promoting adaptation, independence or self-care, they can be held accountable by the public for this particular service.

Activity 2: Medical model

The main home of the medical model is in the hospital system. But hospital care is getting more expensive and there is a trend towards shorter lengths of stay, early discharge, day care, and community care.

Think about whether the medical model is appropriate in this changing healthcare world.

Write a short paper on this and identify a more suitable theory. Refer back to Chapter 4 if you need to remind yourself of the medical model.

Method of selection

Many experienced nurses know what their patients' needs are and this awareness will influence their choice of theory. In previous chapters we have referred many times to tacit knowledge (Polanyi 1958) and how experienced nurses have a 'gut reaction' when it comes to assessing and providing care. But should the selection of a theory be based upon such 'gut reaction' or should nurses be pursuing the best possible empirical evidence to choose the most appropriate theory? The former stance was supported by Mary Silva (1977). She urged nurses to value truths arrived at by intuition and introspection as much as those arrived at by scientific research. In contrast, Aggleton and Chalmers (2000) stressed that preferences must be made on logical grounds. However, in support of Silva's assertion, we are aware that in most cases within nursing, the theory exists before the research to test it is undertaken.

The use of multiple theories

Although the selection within one clinical setting of different theories for different patient groups may be a desirable and recommended strategy (Fawcett 2005), it leads to complications with staff training. It could take a long time for clinical nurses to be educated about a range of theories and how best to employ them in practice. Also, if different theories are used in the same setting there would be problems with the documentation for care planning. Furthermore, using a range of different theories could contribute to communication problems. For example, those staff working across a hospital site such as managers and lecturers would require a high degree of theoretical sophistication. To the uninitiated, such a patient care system may resemble a conceptual 'tower of Babel'. Furthermore, communications within and between members of the multiprofessional team could be hampered by such a strategy and patients who are transferred from ward to ward or from ward to outpatient clinic as their condition changes may have trouble understanding or contributing to their care plans. Fawcett (2005) pointed out that all the successful implementation projects reported in the literature tend to focus on the introduction of only one rather than multiple nursing theories.

Length of patient stay

Time is an important factor when choosing a theory. When one is working within a relatively short time frame, for example, accident and emergency or an acute admission ward, a framework like FANCAP (Walsh 1991) might be suitable. Elsewhere we noted that it has been calculated that to implement Roy's theory correctly would require a care plan of sixteen A4 pages (Miller 1989).

We should consider whether it is right to put patients through a complete care plan assessment and set goals for nursing interventions when they may not be in the clinical setting long enough to receive the interventions or have their care plan goals met. One obvious way to address this is to ensure there is a good discharge plan so that community nurses can pick up the care where the hospital nurses have left off. Nevertheless, if community staff are using a different theory to that used in hospital, the opportunities for confusion and misunderstanding are increased. We asked you to consider the ethical aspects of this example in Activity 1.

Restrictiveness of theories

Each theory is limited by its own assumptions and it follows that no particular one will be able to deal with all eventualities. While nurses may want assurance that a so-called 'right choice' of a theory would eliminate all their patient's care problems, it is possible that the restrictiveness inherent in individual theories may burden nurses with too narrow a perspective. For example, we cannot be criticised for failing to emphasise independence in the activities of daily living (Roper et al. 2000) if the theory we are using stresses the manipulation of stimuli to promote adaptation (Roy 2003). Middle range theories by their nature are even more restrictive. It is possible that a specialist nurse would be using a number of different mid range theories as none on their own will deal with the patient's total needs (see Chapter 4).

Making a wrong choice

Aggleton and Chalmers (2000) believed that the quality of care would be adversely affected by an inappropriate choice of theory, while McKenna (1994) maintained that early closure on an unsuitable theory may stifle creativity. Therefore, mistakenly choosing an unsuitable theory may also have undesirable consequences. An analogy that is often used by metatheorists is that of a map. A map will help direct you to where you want to go and there are different maps depending on your needs. An underground rail map is different to a street map which is also different to a map used by airline pilots. An incorrect choice of a map can get one lost; the same applies to the incorrect choice of a theory. Although an unsuitable choice is regrettable, it is not something that needs to be permanent. Using another analogy, Clark (1986) maintained that if a theory does not fit comfortably, it should be discarded like a pair of ill-fitting shoes.

Staff attitudes

Ersser (2006) claimed that in clinical settings there is a distrust of theories. It is highly likely that the ambivalence felt towards the nursing process has been transferred to theories. Previously, Hawkett (1989) argued that practitioners view theories with suspicion and describe them as 'woolly and impracticable'. Although such negative attitudes do not coincide with McKenna's (1995) research findings, they do influence the selection of theories for practice. It is a truism that if nurses have a view that theories will add more paperwork to their already busy schedule, they will select the simplest theory available and the one that is easy to introduce and manage.

Nursing theories in midwifery

Although several nurse theorists were also midwives, most of the grand theories available have emanated from nursing rather than midwifery. Midgely (1988) found in her study that many midwives used Orem's (1980) theory of nursing. This raises the question of whether nursing theories can be generalised to midwifery or do they have to be altered in the transition? If alteration is required then is the original theoretical status of the theory being compromised? But if it is felt that the grand theories of nursing are broad enough to be applied in most care settings then transference between specialties and health professions may not be an issue.

The suitability of American models

'England and America are two countries separated by a common language.' (George Bernard Shaw 1856–1950)

Although Florence Nightingale (1859) can be credited with being the first nurse theorist, most modern theorists hail from the USA. A question has been posed as to whether their conceptual frameworks are transferable to nursing practice in the UK (Girot 1990). Perhaps there is nothing wrong with nurses from different nations swapping ideas, but the application of one group's practices to the other may not always be appropriate. Because the UK has a different healthcare system to the USA, a different nurse education system and a different culture it is understandable that American theories may not always be the best choice for nursing care elsewhere. But if nurses in different countries continually look towards the USA for conceptual guidance, a manipulative process will have to be employed to ensure their validity within the new health service. In recent years, there have been more theories emanating from the UK and the most popular theory used by British nurses is that of Roper et al. (2000).

Criteria for selecting an appropriate theory

Fawcett (2005: 40) stated that nurses should follow four steps when selecting a nursing theory:

1   Thoroughly analyse and evaluate several nursing theories.
2   Compare the content of each theory with the mission statement of the healthcare institution to determine if the theory is appropriate for use with the population of nursing participants served.

3 Determine if the philosophical claims underpinning each theory are congruent with the philosophy of the nursing department.
4 Select the theory that most closely matches the mission of the healthcare institution and philosophy of the nursing department.

From the foregoing section, the flaws in Fawcett's approach are clear. As we stressed earlier, it would be difficult for busy nurses to analyse and evaluate several nursing theories and, if they could, which ones will they analyse? In addition, points 2 and 3 could be counter-productive. For instance, if the pervading philosophy is the medical model, then the nurses will select a theory that matches this way of working and so maintain the status quo. Therefore, there is a danger that Fawcett's four-stage approach to selecting a theory will not lead to innovative and creative ways of thinking and practising.

The theoretical literature in nursing abounds with frameworks drawn up for theory analysis and evaluation (Meleis 1985, 1991, 1997, 2007; Fawcett 2005; Alligood & Marriner Tomey 2006; Chinn & Kramer 2004). In essence, most are made up of features and topics which theories have in common. These features are condensed within a scheme and form a means of comparison between theories. We will deal with this in more detail in Chapter 9. Frameworks have another use in that they may be used as a checklist for selecting an appropriate theory.

Origins of the theory

If a theory has its basis in the 'know-how' of practice (Rhyl 1963), it may be more attractive to hard pressed clinical nurses. In contrast, a theory that was formulated by academic 'armchair theorists' who based their work on reasoning alone, may be unattractive to clinical nurses. Therefore, when selecting a theory nurses should explore the research and practice origins of those that do exist. If a theory is neither reliable nor valid then the practice being guided by that theory will be suspect. Therefore, theories that emerge inductively from clinical practice rather than being formulated from the minds of theorists may have more credibility with clinical nurses. It is of course possible to identify a theory that was developed through 'retroduction'. From Chapter 6 readers will remember that this is where both induction and deduction played a part. For instance, Peplau (1962) studied the phenomenon of interpersonal relations over many years and began to develop her theory deductively through the influence of Harry Stack Sullivan's interpersonal relations theory (1953) and inductively through reflecting on her clinical experience in psychiatric nursing. This gives clinical nurses the best of both worlds – the theory has clinical credibility and is based on good science.

Type of patient

When considering theories for practice, nurses should not be too concerned with which theory is popular in their country or region; rather they should be concerned with which is best for the needs of their patients. Therefore, the most appropriate choice of any theory must be based on the nurses' knowledge of their patient population. The theory must also be general enough to deal with the many diverse situations the nurse comes across when dealing with a heterogeneous group of patients.

Healthcare setting

This criterion is related to the previous one but concentrates on contextual factors in the nursing situation. Glaser and Strauss stated that 'theory must fit the substantive area in which it is to be used' (Glaser & Strauss 1967: 237). Earlier in this chapter we likened theories to maps that guide our practice; we require a different map to suit the specific terrain in which we find ourselves. Therefore, staff in different clinical settings should select a theory depending on the fit of that theory to the function of that setting.

Parsimony/simplicity

'Occam's razor' states that 'the simplest theory is to be selected from among all other theories that fit the facts as we know them' (William of Occam, 1300–49). This traditional belief is synonymous with the modern idea of 'parsimony'. Elsewhere we stated that parsimony dictates that a good theory is one that is stated in the simplest terms possible. There are complex idealistic theories such as that of Rogers (1970) and there are less complex but realistic theories such as that of Henderson (1966). There is little reason to select the former if the latter will suit the clinical requirements just as well.

Understandability

Although this concept relates closely to parsimony, it merits separate consideration. A theory must be easily understood if it is to get the support of busy nurses. How can a nurse use a theory if she cannot understand it? Jackson (1986) wondered what uses elaborate lines and circles were if nurses cannot employ them to guide their practice. Nonetheless, in case we become over-critical of the complexity of theory, we should take cognisance of the fact that a theory must have an element of complexity to be significant. Bronowski (2005) stated in *The Ascent of Man* that the language of science cannot be freed from ambiguity any more than poetry can. Furthermore, the Irish orator Edmund Burke (1729–97) stated that a thing may look specious in theory, and yet be ruinous in practice – a thing may look evil in theory, yet in practice be excellent.

Activity 3: Understandability and jargon

We have noticed, over the years, examples of anti-intellectualism among many nurses. They complain about the big words and jargon used in nursing theories and nursing research. However, they appear to be enthusiastically fluent when it comes to knowing and reciting the long and complex names of certain diseases, medical interventions and pharmaceutical products.

Take a few minutes to consider why this is the case and what can be done to change this. Discuss with your fellow students whether this is a realistic observation of nursing behaviour or simply a biased perception on our part.

Miller (1989) maintained that, when selecting a theory, the relevance to practice is central. She suggested that the person who is choosing the theory should seek answers to the following questions (Miller 1989: 47):

- Does the theory have direct relevance for the way in which nursing is practised?
- Does the theory describe real or 'ought-to-be' care?
- Has its assumptions and propositions been tried and tested?
- Does it deal with the resources which are necessary for good care?
- Does it guide the use of the nursing process?
- Does it provide practising nurses with good direction for clinical actions?

- Are the concepts within the theory too abstract to be applied in practice?
- Is the language of the theory easy to understand?
- Does the theory coincide with the practising nurse's 'know-how' knowledge?

Paradigms as a basis for choice

In Chapter 5 we pointed out that every nursing theory has its roots in one or more of the following paradigms: systems, interactional, developmental and behavioural. These 'worldviews' could help nurses make some preliminary decisions about the type of theory that is most appropriate for their work. This seems sensible as nurses who espouse an interactional approach to caring would be unlikely to select a systems theory to guide their practice (Maloney 1984).

Practitioners' values and beliefs as a basis for choice

As nurses we all have a personal perception in our minds regarding the central components of our profession. This is based upon our attitudes, values and beliefs and is borne out of the education and experience we have been exposed to over a number of years.

It is a given that clinical practice varies according to the beliefs and attitudes of the nurse giving the care. These values and beliefs have been referred to as the nurse's implicit nursing theory (McKenna 1997). Previously, McFarlane wrote:

> 'Most (practitioners) have a rough picture of practice which includes ideas about the nature and role of the patient and the nurse, the environment . . . in which practice takes place, and the major field of function, i.e. health care and the nature of action.' (McFarlane 1986: 3)

It follows therefore that all nurses have a personal theory that they use to guide their practice. These personal theories incorporate assumptions concerning the four metaparadigm elements of nursing, health, person and environment (see Chapter 5). Therefore, nurses can use these informal personal nursing theories to help them select suitable formal theories.

If asked, most nurses are able to reveal these personal theories; they can identify their views on what nursing, health, environment and person are. However, in the reality of the practice situation these are seldom articulated. Consequently, they are mostly hidden in the nurse's mind rather than being made explicit (Clarke 1986).

Some of the problems with this approach to selecting a nursing theory have already been identified above. The main one is the perpetuation of the theoretical status quo. If the nurse's personal theory is based only on being educated and experienced in the medical model, this will reflect her choice of theory. There are other limitations to matching a personal theory with an established one. For instance, Bishop (1986) feared that these 'personal guides to practice' may be incomplete, unproved, inconsistent and muddled.

Furthermore, the internationally recognised nursing theories are by no means 'value free'. They too were initially formulated around the personal views and preferences of their architects. By selecting these nursing theories, practising nurses may simply be exchanging their own biased view with that of another. Nonetheless, in an era where nursing theories are often perceived to be unpopular, selecting one that best reflects their perception of nursing may be the most effective. After all, nurses will have difficulty 'signing up' to a nursing theory if it does not coincide with their deep-rooted views of what they believe nursing is.

A strategy for choice

From the above discussion we would suggest that every nurse has a personal theory pertaining to how they view the metaparadigm components. You will recall in the previous chapter that published theories also have statement and views of the metaparadigm. Hence, practitioners can choose a theory that best reflects their beliefs and values related to these elements (McKenna 1997). This is an essential prerequisite if the theory is to fit the reality of practice. When considering the selection of a theory for psychiatric nursing Mansfield (1980) wrote:

'Although it is advisable to practice what we preach, it is difficult, if not impossible to practice what we could not preach from the heart.' (Mansfield 1980: 34)

As alluded to above, Fawcett (2005) maintained that the beliefs a nurse holds about the person, the environment, health and nursing will direct her to look for a theory congruent with these beliefs. Therefore she can compare the content of theories with her beliefs and select the one that closely matches them.

As mentioned above, if nurses cannot accept how some concepts are treated within a particular theory they should reject that theory and choose another whose concepts would be more compatible with their own. In this way congruence will be reached between the nurse's clinical orientation and a recognised theory. The final choice will indicate for nurses what they have always believed about their work but could not articulate in as clear and distinct manner as the selected theory could.

Who should select the theory?

The literature is unclear about this, and merely suggests that practitioners be involved (Aggleton & Chalmers 2000).

Adam outlined some helpful suggestions (Adam 1980: 82):

- A committee or group make their choice from existing theories.
- Every concerned individual participates in a comparative study of several theories.
- An entire group develops its own specific theory.
- A group chooses an existing theory, but plans to develop their own.
- The group takes 'bits and pieces' from several theories to form an 'eclectic' theory.

Adam pointed out that although the first two methods are lengthy processes, in the end the change will be more lasting if every concerned individual has been party to the decision-making process. He maintained that a decision imposed by others often means a short-lived allegiance among those that have to implement it.

More controversial is the suggestion that perhaps the nurse manager of each clinical unit should select the most relevant theory. This may indeed be a valid nomination considering that Kitson (1984) identified the ward sister as possessing the most knowledge and influence regarding clinical work orientation and practical expertise.

There is a general absence of literature suggesting that the patient be involved in the theory selection process. This is strange considering the emphasis on the patient as a partner in care. But when selecting a theory, the beliefs and values of the most important person concerned, the recipient of care, cannot be ignored. However, if nursing theories are viewed as confusing to many nurses, would patients not find them even more confusing? If the answer is yes then one can see why there has been little evidence of partnership between nurses and patients in the selection of a theory.

Borrowed or home-grown theory?

An important issue to consider when selecting a theory for nursing is whether we should borrow theories from other disciplines. Over 40 years ago Wald and Leonard (1964) argued that if practitioners continued to borrow theories from other disciplines, research problems based upon these theories will be phrased as questions that have little to do with nursing. For instance, using and testing sociological theories within nursing may do more for the knowledge base of sociology than for nursing. Wald and Leonard called for the development of nursing theories rather than trying to make borrowed theories fit. But is this too narrow a view? Should we not use whatever theory fits the patient problem and can best guide practice?

A panel of well-known theorists rejected Meleis's call for nurses to theorise with multidisciplinary colleagues (Huch 1995). They still maintained that we should adhere to the goal of developing theory specifically for nursing practice. Perhaps there is some merit in this suggestion. Compared to sociology, psychology, medicine, law and many other professions, nursing is still a relatively new discipline. It requires a body of knowledge pertaining to its practice. We would however suggest that the choice should not be either/or. Nurses should formulate their own theories but they should also use and develop theories with other disciplines.

To a large extent this corresponds with the picture in other professions. Social workers for instance began with an adherence to the medical model, only to supplant it with theories of their own as their discipline evolved.

In many instances, nurses borrow theories but do not bother to adapt them. This often results in theory that is incomplete and poorly representative of nursing. To be useful, such borrowed knowledge must be reformulated and revalidated to suit the particular problems and needs of our discipline. For example, psychological or organisational theories are not unique to nursing; however, how they are used and the perspective employed can be unique. Yet, because borrowed theories may need to undergo intensive reworking to fit nursing's unique perspective, borrowing may not be as simple a process as it first appears and we could end up with an invalid and unreliable hybrid.

We should, however, not be worried about ownership; theories belong to the scientific community at large, not to one particular discipline. Discovery does not confer the right of ownership. A note of caution: nurses should be careful to avoid the temptation of borrowing from other disciplines without first investigating what those theories have done for those disciplines. If a sociological theory of family care is rejected by sociologists, it may be foolish for nurses to borrow it for their practice unless careful consideration is given to why it was rejected by its parent discipline.

Dickoff and James (1971) took a different view. They asked 'why is borrowing so wrong?' and argued that it is the output for practice that is relevant, not some notion of ownership or a contribution to a unique body of knowledge. They called for 'this foolish emphasis on idiosyncrasy in concept, method or definition' to be abandoned for more relevant concerns of practice.

The term 'borrowed' suggests that it will be returned to where it came from. In this case nursing may adapt a borrowed theory and improve upon it. As a result the adapted theory could bring new perspectives for its parent discipline.

It may not be long before other healthcare disciplines begin to borrow theories developed by nurses. In fact, there is some evidence to suggest that occupational therapists and physiotherapists are borrowing and reformulating nursing theories (e.g. self-care and activity-of-living theories) for their practices.

We maintain that there is nothing wrong with selecting a theory from another discipline if it can shed new light or provide a different beneficial perspective on the provision of patient care. There is no reason why nurses should 're-invent the wheel'. The important question is whether selecting a 'borrowed' theory brings with it benefits for nursing, nurses and the people who rely on us for care.

Summary

Because the choice of a theory will affect how patients are assessed and how care is planned and delivered, selection should not be a process which nurses take lightly. This chapter identified several issues that must be taken into consideration when an appropriate theory is to be chosen. It outlined a range of selection criteria which readers may find useful. The issues of who should make the choice and how this should be done were also addressed. In essence, there are many selection approaches available and nurses should consider these carefully. Not to do so could waste a lot of time and choose an inappropriate theory to guide practice.

Remember, theories are like maps and we require a different one depending on the terrain in which we are working. The days should be over when managers and tutors choose theories for practice. Patients or their representatives should work alongside nurses in the selection process. If this occurs, the selected theory will be a realistic reflection of what those in practice see as important for quality of care, and nurses will be more likely to use it enthusiastically and appropriately.

Web addresses

Readers may find the following web addresses useful:

http://www.sandiego.edu/academics/nursing/theory/
http://www.enursescribe.com/nurse_theorists.htm
http://www.healthsci.clayton.edu/eichelberger/nursing.htm

Research-Based Theories or Theory-Based Research?

'In Research the Horizon recedes as we advance . . . and research is always incomplete.'

Isaac Casaubon, M. Pattison (1813–84)

Outline of content

This chapter outlines the relationship between research and theory. It deals with how theory is generated by research, tested by research, and evaluated by research. It also highlights how theory can help frame a research study. Furthermore, the chapter looks at how the levels of theory as identified by Dickoff and James can be linked to research approaches. The text guides the reader through the process of identifying an interesting occurrence in practice and taking it through to theory development and testing.

The relationship between theory, practice and research is one of mutual support and development (Young et al. 2001). Theories often emerge from practice, are tested by research and are returned to practice unchanged, adapted or strengthened. You will recall that phenomena are things, events or situations that you perceive through your senses. Nurses continually notice phenomena in their daily work with patients. Some ignore such phenomena, believing them to be unimportant, while others give considerable thought to why the phenomena are there and what causes them to appear.

For instance, suppose Trish Reid, an oncology nurse, notices that children who are in hospital for chemotherapy appear less stressed and agitated when their parents are present. She sees this as an interesting phenomenon and seeks confirmation of her observations with colleagues. They too notice this and observe that it appears to be related to the child's age and length of time in hospital.

Trish decides to investigate the phenomenon further and researches it as part of her master's degree. She uses a qualitative survey design where she interviews children on the oncology unit, oncology nurses and parents. The data collected support her hunch that this is an important phenomenon and a theory begins to take shape. She calls it the 'parent support' theory and it postulates that children between the ages of 6 and 12 who have a diagnosis of cancer and are being given chemotherapy show almost no signs of stress and anxiety when their parents are with them compared to when they are not. The children most affected are those who have been undergoing inpatient chemotherapy for a least a week.

In this example, the 'parent support' theory emerged from practice as a middle range theory. We will expand below on how a phenomenon emerges and how it can be given a name to make it a concept and how different concepts form propositions which in turn form theory. Trish and her supervisor decide to publish her research in a cancer nursing journal. As a result of the publication a nurse researcher in Australia decides to test the theory to see if it can be verified or refuted when applied to children in a number of oncology units in Sydney.

Activity 1: Phenomena to theory?

You will now know how phenomena identified in a nurse's daily work can be thought about and labelled as concepts that can then be linked as propositions that can form a theory.

Think of an event that you have noticed in your practice or clinical setting. Consider this phenomenon and in a one-page account, take it through the same process that Trish Reid did.

From Chapter 3 you will recall that Popper (1965) supported carrying out research to refute theory. You may also remember that we used the analogy of a kite. Another way to visualise this process is to consider a theory to be a paper boat. You construct the paper boat and you see if it floats. The first time you push it out into the pond it floats and so the boat has been well constructed. You try putting small weights in the boat to see if it still floats and you try to make the water choppier. If the boat remains floating after all these tests then it has done everything that was required of it. However, it is also possible that after two or three tests the boat sinks (the theory is refuted). A great deal can be learned from its sinking that could lead to the construction of a better and stronger boat.

The same principle applies to the testing of Trish Reid's 'parent support' theory. The Sydney researchers could replicate her qualitative study. Alternatively, they could test the theory deductively using a quantitative approach. They could do this by asking children who are similar in age and length of stay to those interviewed by Trish to complete stress and anxiety tests. This could be done when their parents are present and when they are absent. The results, like those with the paper boat, will show that the theory is either verified or refuted. If the former, the Australian team of researchers can publish the results showing that their research in Sydney upholds the 'parent support' theory. They may also make recommendations to strengthen the theory and these could be taken up by other researchers in other parts of the world. Over time, the theory becomes established – until of course another test refutes it. However, if it is never refuted, the theory finds its way into nursing textbooks and initiatives involving parents in the care of their hospitalised children with cancer. In time it becomes part of established practice. In summary, the 'parent support' theory has emerged from practice, has been tested and has returned to inform practice. This reciprocal relationship between theory, research and practice is how science can be developed in nursing and how theory can lead to improvements in patient care.

From the foregoing example you will see that research does two main things: it generates theory or it tests theory. Jacox (1974) stated that research without theory was analogous to a team of bricklayers, each making a brick in isolation from other bricklayers and no blueprint to follow. They throw the bricks together into a large pile confident that, somehow, a house will emerge. Similarly, Trish Reid could easily have ignored the phenomenon she observed and failed to see the propositional relationship between the concepts – children with cancer, their parents, their age, their length of stay, anxiety and stress. To use Jacox's analogy, these would just be disregarded bricks. Therefore, without theory, the knowledge Trish Reid obtained would be a mass of data and observations with no coherence or understanding.

New theory generated from practice will lead to new research studies which will lead to new knowledge for practice. In turn, new knowledge presents us with new facts which encourage us to develop theories to explain these facts. Unfortunately, too often practice is carried out without being guided by research or theory. Furthermore, studies continue to be undertaken which are descriptive and poorly linked to theory.

Meleis (2007) stated that researchers often view theorists as 'ivory tower' philosophers who dream up ideas unconnected with practice or research. Similarly, theorists view researchers as investigators who focus on small research projects to confirm or not confirm disconnected propositions that do not add up to theory. Such research has limited usefulness. The end product of research is poor if it does not provide theory to help describe or explain phenomena or help practising nurses to prescribe interventions and predict outcomes.

Earlier we introduced you to the seminal work, 'A theory of theories' by Dickoff and James (1968). The authors stated that research is for the sake of theory and theory is for the sake of practice and that theory produced without research has little hope of viability. Research, they say is pointless unless done (a) in the context of theory and (b) with a clear realisation of what it can contribute to theory.

At the outset of a study, researchers should ask themselves the following questions:

- Is this study generating new theory?
- Is it testing existing theory?
- Is this theory worth generating or testing?
- What effect will it have on practice?
- Will the research contribute to the scientific body of knowledge?

Nursing has been criticised over the years for the large number of grand theories that have been generated by 'armchair' theorists. These are nurses who through reasoning rather than active research have developed theories. Not only were these not generated through research, most were not tested by research either. In fact, it could be argued that the concepts and propositions within them were so broad in scope that it would not be possible to test them. It is a truism that if nurses are taught theories that have no basis in research, the nursing care based on these theories could have no positive effect on patients. Teachers and managers who promulgate such theories must be aware of the ethical implications of doing so. Their implementation in practice in an unquestioning manner may do a great deal of harm and may become just as much a ritual as the habitual carrying out of existing unsubstantiated routines.

Activity 2: Propositions from grand theory

By now you will know that all theories are made up of concepts and statements (propositions) linking them together in some way. Grand theories such as those of Roper et al., Orem, Roy, and so on are also composed of these elements.

> For this exercise, select one theory with which you are familiar or one from a textbook. Identify one or two propositions in that theory and write a short report on how you would go about testing whether the prepositional relationship was valid.

For many years now, research approaches in nursing have been divided into two main camps. There are hypothesis-testing studies where, through deductive testing, the object is to create explanatory and practice theories (what Dickoff and James referred to as 'situation relating' and 'situation producing' theories). In the past such research was labelled positivism or empiricism (see Chapter 3). In contrast, qualitative research uses induction where the object is to create descriptive and exploratory theories. Trish Reid used this approach to create the 'parent support' theory.

Chalmers (1989) pointed out that positivist approaches to theory development mimic work in the natural sciences where researchers are motivated to discover universal laws. In nursing this may be a fruitless search because such laws may be untenable in human science. Quantitative and qualitative research may be differentiated by where the theory is in the research process. In qualitative research the theory is the product and emerges (possibly not fully formed) at the end of the study. In contrast, in quantitative research the theory is present at the beginning of the study and the researcher formulates hypotheses from its propositions, and tests these to see if the theory's propositions can be refuted or verified. In theory-generating research the researcher seeks to identify a phenomenon, discover its characteristics and formulate propositions; in theory-testing research the investigator seeks to develop evidence about hypotheses derived from the theory's propositions.

Stevens Barnum (1998) failed to recognise the existence of research that is not linked in some way to theory. She maintained that theory directs research, research corrects theory, and corrected theory directs more research. In contrast, Chinn and Kramer (2004) argued that there are two main types of research: theory-linked research and theory-isolated research. They concede that both can be of excellent quality and can contribute to new knowledge, but because the former is conducted within the framework of theory it has greater potential for developing new understanding. Theory-linked research is related to the generation or the testing of theory while, by definition, theory-isolated research has no discernible theoretical connection. In both types of research, questions may come from the imagination, from work experience, from a hunch or from a number of other sources.

In our experience there are four possible linkages between research and theory (McKenna 1997):

- Research generates theory inductively from practice (theory-generating research, TGR).
- Research tests theory deductively in practice (theory-testing research, TTR).
- Theory guides the research project (theory-framed research, TFR).
- Research evaluates the use of theory in practice (theory-evaluating research, TER).

Theory-generating research

Jacox (1974) identified three empiricist type stages to the inductive generation of theory.

- The researcher must identify the phenomena of interest within the field of study and specify, define and classify the concepts used in describing these phenomena.
- The researcher develops statements or propositions that propose how two or more concepts are related.
- The researcher specifies how the propositions are related to each other in a systematic way.

Elsewhere in this book we have illustrated the difference between grand theory, middle range theory and practice theory (see Chapter 4). Grand theories are very broad and in most cases have not been generated through research. Mostly they have been developed through reasoning based upon experience. This included the work of Orem (1980) and Henderson (1966). However, such an approach to theory development is not new. You will recall that Freud created his psychoanalytic theories without ever carrying out any empirical research.

In contrast, middle range and practice theories have their base in research. Speaking generally for science, Laudan (1977) stated that theoretical progress in a discipline is often measured by the number and the quality of the theories developed by its scholars. Therefore, the most useful outcome of nursing research is the number of meaningful theories that impact positively on the health and wellbeing of patients, their families and communities. TGR contributes significantly to the growth of such theories.

When little is known about clinical phenomena, TGR research is conducted for the purpose of their discovery and exploration. The resultant theories are normally generated inductively by researchers who realise that within nursing practice there lie a large number of phenomena awaiting observation and description. Because the research eventually leads to inductively formulated theory, TGR may be referred to as the research-then-theory approach to knowledge development.

Identifying the clinical setting as the seedbed for theory, Dickoff and James (1992) claimed that since nursing practice predates nursing research it makes a sound foundation for theorising. Furthermore, if nurse researchers are to be expert in TGR they must work in partnership with clinical staff who can provide them with research-worthy phenomena of specific interest to patient care.

Chinn and Kramer (2004) pointed out that when attempting to generate theory the researcher enters the research setting with as open a mind as possible in order to see new relationships between phenomena. However, we all have our own conceptual 'baggage' which we bring to new situations and so this is not always an easy process. Furthermore, interesting researchable phenomena may be perceived by clinical nurses with years of experience as humdrum and ordinary. Therefore, researchers and the clinical staff they work with should be acutely aware of the possibilities that phenomena have for theory generation but also of their possible biases.

Approaches to theory generation

A grounded theory approach involves the simultaneous collection of data, coding, categorising observations and forming concepts and relationships based on the data. In grounded theory the researcher begins to write impressions about the meaning of the data as they are collected (Glaser & Strauss 1967).

Ethnography has its basis in social anthropology. The researcher seeks to become involved in the setting, to experience the phenomenon first hand and to soak up the concepts which are important in describing that phenomenon.

Phenomenology is designed to describe the subjective lived experiences of people and to comprehend the essence and meanings that people place on these experiences. The experiences cannot be observed, they can only be directly accessible to the person who has the experience.

Phenomenology results in narratives where the participant has told their story about their lived experience. Grounded theory results in new or existing concepts joined together by propositional statements. Ethnography results in observations that lead to new ways of viewing phenomena. Regardless of approach, findings are usually presented in the form of concepts and propositions which form the basis for a theory. While the end result of TGR is often middle range theory, the following grand theories were developed using interpretative qualitative approaches: Parse (1981), Patterson and Zderad (1976) and Watson (1985).

The research process in theory-generating research

In TGR, the clinical problem, the research questions and the research purpose need to be stated in advance. According to Chinn and Kramer (2004) research hypotheses may also be used. However, more commonly, research questions or problem statements are enough to guide the investigation.

In TGR the data are collected by direct (physical) observation or indirect observation (interviews/focus groups). In addition, because of their inherent theoretical bias, research instruments such as structured questionnaires or scales may not be very useful in TGR. Where the aim is to collect narrative data, care must be taken to ensure that the approaches used will elicit the type of unbiased responses which are required.

Because the sample must link the theoretical aspects of the study to the reality of practice the following assumption is made: there is some phenomenon or event happening in the real world that will be evident if I observe these events or this particular group of people. Furthermore, this event or group of people is sufficiently like other events or groups of people who have this experience.

Strange as it may seem, a time series with comparison group can also be used for the qualitative generation of theory. For example, if researchers were studying the experiences of hospitalisation of persons with mental health problems, they might take a longitudinal approach whereby qualitative data are collected before, during and after the hospitalisation. At the same time they might identify other groups of patients with similar problems who are being treated in the community. The comparison would tell the researcher if aspects of the phenomena of anxiety and self-esteem were unique to one care setting or another. These data would contribute to the development of theory related to the hospitalisation experience.

In TGR the analysis involves identifying themes and categories that emanate from the data. The researcher proposes concepts generated from the data and, if the evidence supports them, theoretical propositions. In most TGR projects the concepts and propositions may not be evident until the results of the data analysis are presented.

The discussion and conclusions focus on the theoretical significance of the study. In TGR though, the conclusions centre on the newly

Table 8.1 Types of propositional statements developed through TGR.

Descriptive proposition: there is a relationship between x and y Directional proposition: there is a positive relationship between x and y Concurrent proposition: if x, then also y Sequential proposition: if x, then later y Deterministic proposition: if x, then always y, if no interfering conditions Probabilistic (stochastic) proposition: if x, then probably y Necessary proposition: if x, and only if x, then y Substitutional proposition: if x_1, but also x_2, then y Sufficient proposition: if x then y, regardless of anything else Contingent proposition: if x, then y, in the presence of c

discovered concepts and relevant propositions. These are often immediately useful in practice because of their grounding in the experience or setting from which the theory was generated. Table 8.1 summarises the types of proposition that may emanate from TGR.

The next step in TGR is diagramming or putting the concepts and propositions into diagrammatic form. Diagramming is done after the concepts, definitions and propositions have been identified and propositions have been hierarchically ordered by level of abstraction (Fawcett & Downs 1992). Within the diagram the existence of a relationship is denoted by an unbroken line. For connecting concepts, an arrowhead at one end indicates an asymmetrical relationship and an arrowhead at both ends indicates a symmetrical relationship. A positive relationship is denoted by a + sign and a negative relationship is denoted by a – sign. A question mark may be used if the direction is unclear (see Figure 8.1).

In a robust TGR study there is a comprehensive literature review pertaining to the phenomenon being studied, the method employed is clear and the resultant concepts and propositional statements are specified. Where possible the researcher should also make clear what type of propositional statements have been generated and illustrate by diagram the relationship in terms of existence, direction and symmetry. Some of the above propositions may also be stated as researchable hypotheses. In this way TGR is opening up an opportunity for TTR to take place (see Figure 8.3).

In TGR, the findings may:

- lead to the formulation of a new theory
- lead to the support of an existing theory
- lead to a rejection of an existing theory
- lead to an existing theory being adapted or revised.

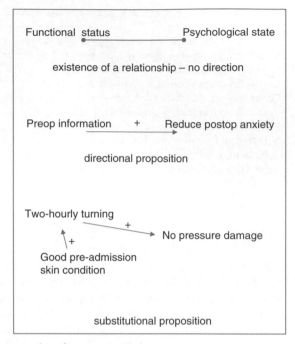

Figure 8.1 Examples of propositional diagramming.

Theory-testing research

Because those who undertake TTR propose an *a priori* theory from which hypotheses are derived and then verified or refuted through research, TTR could be referred to as the theory-then-research process.

In TTR a theory exists and research is undertaken to establish its validity. However, this is factually incorrect. A theory may have many propositions and what the researcher does is to turn the propositions into hypotheses and test them. Furthermore, they may not test all the propositions. For the purposes of this chapter we will refer to this process as theory testing.

The research methods in theory-testing studies are designed to ascertain how accurately the theory depicts real-world phenomena and their relationships. For a theory to be testable you need:

- concepts that describe the phenomena of interest;
- theoretical and operational definitions of these concepts;
- propositions – links between the concepts that describe, explain or predict phenomena.

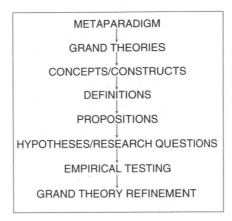

Figure 8.2 A typical theory-testing process.

As mentioned above, theory testing normally involves a deductive approach where hypotheses are tested using randomised controlled trials, experimental or quasi-experimental approaches. Research questions can also be used to test a theory; this usually takes place within a correlational design. The concepts within the research questions or hypotheses are derived from the theory. Figure 8.2 shows one such theory-testing process (adapted from Moody 1990). Please note that the process illustrated is not necessary linear – it may be iterative.

The research process

In TTR the research purpose, the research problem and the hypotheses/or research questions are designed to show the relationships between the theory and the research study and these are formulated in advance of conducting the study. Previous studies based upon the theory form a substantial part of the literature review. The review also includes a critique of alternative theories shown to be relevant to the study's central purpose. Furthermore, the literature review indicates how the study was conceived and why the specific propositional relationships within the theory are being tested. There should also be a critical review of existing research that relates to the topic.

In TTR the data are collected by direct (physical observation) or indirect observation (interviews and self completion tools such as questionnaires and scales). Psychometric properties of the data collection tools such as reliability and validity should be given serious consideration. The sample and population must be carefully considered and invariably statistical power analysis is used in deciding the sample size.

In TTR, the analysis focuses on whether the data present sufficient evidence to support or reject the hypotheses or answer the research questions. Conclusions are then made regarding the empirical adequacy of the theory.

The reasons why a theory is verified or refuted may not always be obvious, but knowledge and understanding have been increased and possible false leads have been eradicated (Stevens Barnum 1998). Strange as it may seem, theory testing research may actually lead to theory generation. Because of the insight gained through the research, the basis for a new theory may be formed.

As with the kite or paper boat analogies, a theory is a description or explanation for phenomena until a better one comes along.

Moody (1990) argued that nursing must:

- develop innovative strategies for theory testing through research;
- encourage nurse scholars to generate testable hypotheses deduced from the underlying assumptions and propositions of existing nursing theories;
- organise multiple site studies at national and international levels where several investigators can focus on systematic testing of hypotheses from nursing theories;
- identify criteria for theory testing in nursing research and nursing theory courses;
- collaborate in national and international research endeavours with practitioners who are engaged in implementing nursing theories in clinical areas.

However, some theories are not testable because of ethical considerations. For instance, while theories may be formulated on sleep deprivation in children or on the starvation of pregnant women, it would be unethical to test them in practice. There are other reasons for theories not being testable. It is well known that the technology and methods required to test Einstein's (1879–1955) theory of relativity ($e = mc^2$) were not available until many years after it was developed.

TTR is linked to the traditional positivist/empirical science approach to knowledge development where measurement is extremely important. However, over 35 years ago Rosemary Ellis (1970) asserted that if nurse researchers limited themselves to that which can be measured they ran the risk of studying trivia or issues tangential to nursing.

To conclude this section; there has been a great deal written about the necessity to test theories of relevance to nursing so as to provide evidence of the validity and accuracy of their concepts and propositions. However, little progress has been made towards this goal either by the theorists themselves, researchers, or by those nurses who use them in practice. Not to test theory would have consequences for the

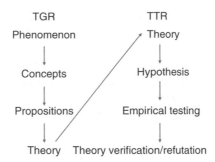

Figure 8.3 The developmental relationship between theory generation and theory testing.

quality of care because of the implications of nurses using a theory of dubious validity to underpin the care of patients. In TTR, the findings may:

* confirm the validity of the theory
* refute the validity of the theory
* lead to the theory being adapted or revised
* lead to the formulation of a new theory.

Figure 8.3 shows how TGR is related to TTR. TGR uses induction to generate theory and TTR uses deduction to test theory. When both are used in the same study this is called retroduction (see Chapter 3).

Theory-framed research

In TFR researchers may not necessarily be generating theory or testing theoretical propositions. Rather, the theory is used to frame the study and provide it with a focus. So important is the theoretical framework that researchers could more easily dispense with the physical operations of a study than the framework which gives meaning to all the research activity. The same methods could be used in a different study and give different outcomes if the conceptual framework were changed.

When used as a framework to structure a study, a theory can:

* give direction to the investigation
* abstract, summarise and order research findings
* relate the study to previous research.

More specifically, Moody (1990) stated that when a theory acts as a framework for research it serves to provide parameters for the study, guides data collection and provides a perspective for interpreting the data so that the researcher is able to weave together the findings in a meaningful pattern. When a study is placed within such a theoretical context the theory guides the research process from the research questions through design, analysis and interpretation to the conclusions. Researchers should identify the theoretical framework at the beginning of the study, however tentative it may seem. It is this theoretical framework which determines what questions will be addressed by the study and how the data will be collected.

For example, if you were investigating how students' examination results are affected by the introduction of an e-learning course you may use a learning theory to frame your study. Similarly, if the research topic is how families cope when their loved one has a stroke you may use 'transitional' theory (Meleis 2007) or 'uncertainty in illness' theory (Mishel 1990). Another example is using the 'end of life' theory (Ruland & Moore 1998) to frame a study on palliative care or the 'theory of planned action' (Ajzen 1998) if you were studying an aspect of health promotion.

However, the selected theory must be relevant and used in a meaningful way. Too often we have seen students introduce the theoretical framework at the beginning of a study to lend the research report some theoretical credibility. In many instances the theory is not referred to again and was, in reality, merely 'theoretical window dressing'. A potentially more serious problem relates to the inappropriate selection of a theory to frame the study. Such a choice may lead to premature commitment to a particular theory with the result that theoretical and clinical vision is restricted. For instance, a family support theory developed by a social anthropologist in the Brazilian rain forest may not be appropriate when applied to a study on the effects of family therapy in the UK. Similarly, a theory that focuses on self-care may miss patients who do not want to be independent.

A theoretical framework used to structure a research study may take on an agenda-setting role, bringing with it inherent biases. Reed (1989) put it very well when she stated that the conceptual nets cast out by researchers could be used to catch fish only of their liking. Like all good investigators nurse researchers should ask 'why' when they start a study and the answer should contain a relevance to nursing. Controversially, Fawcett (2006) argued that in research that pertains to nursing practice, the theory framing the study should be a nursing one. However, because of the relatively short history of nursing theories this may be too narrow a focus. A better suggestion would be that whatever theory the nurse researcher uses to frame the study it should lead to new knowledge that will have a positive impact for the profession and how it practises.

We see a theoretical framework like a 'red thread' that goes through the study linking the various parts of it together such as the literature review, the methodology, the findings and conclusions. It forms a framework on which the study hangs. For instance, if a study was focusing on the development of advanced practitioners in nursing, the researcher could use role theory (Biddle & Thomas 1966) to frame the research. From Chapter 4 you will recall the concepts that make up role theory. In such a TFR study, one would expect to see reference in the literature review to role conflict, role overlap, role norms, role set, role stress and role confusion. The questions asked in the questionnaire or interview schedule would also reflect these concepts. The findings and discussion sections could also be structured with subheadings from role theory. In such a study, role theory is not being generated or tested; rather it is being used almost as a theoretical skeleton for the research.

In TFR, the findings may:

- contribute indirectly to establishing the worth of the theory as a template for the study
- ensure that the study is focused
- lead to a rejection of an existing theory as a guide for a research study
- lead to an existing theory being adapted or revised as a guide for a research study.

Theory-evaluating research

There is the potential for confusion between TER and TTR. However, there are significant differences. Because of their broad scope, grand theories cannot easily be tested and the best we can do is to evaluate their application to see if they have any noticeable effect. Holden (1990) agreed, stating that while it may not be possible to research the underlying assumptions and propositions of some nursing theories, it is possible to scrutinise certain aspects of nursing care affected by their introduction.

In the UK many hospital managers dictated that nurses should use a grand theory to guide practice. This order from on high meant that theories such as Henderson (1966) Orem (1980), and Roy (1980) were being 'shoe-horned' into practice without reference to their suitability and without a sound knowledge of the theory. In most cases the theory was used to structure the assessment of the patient on admission and it had no further application thereafter. In a small number of instances it was used to assess, plan and guide nursing actions. A perusal of the research literature shows that many of these theories were not evaluated with regard to whether they had a positive, negative or neutral effect on patient care. TER focuses on such an evaluation. It is not testing the hypotheses that are derived from the theory's propositions but what impact the theory has through being used in practice. We will discuss the evaluation of theories in greater detail in Chapter 9. In the meantime a short overview here will suffice.

Despite the fact that nursing theories have been taught in the USA and the UK for some years now, the amount of empirical research concerning their effect on nurse learning is conspicuous by its scarcity.

In 1991, Salanders and Dietz-Omar reported the results of an American survey into whether nurses believed nursing theories helped them in clinical decision-making. Data were collected at three points in time: prior to taking a nursing theory course, on completion of the course, and two years later. At the first data collection point respondents were neutral in their responses, neither agreeing nor disagreeing when asked if nursing theories provided a guide for their clinical decision-making. However, at the two latter data collection points the respondents believed that nursing theories did indeed provide such a guide.

Although Salanders and Dietz-Omar (1991) gave detailed statistical results in their research, they omitted to include all aspects relevant to methodology. Without this information one cannot judge the entire relevance or applicability of their findings.

After undertaking a comprehensive trawl of the literature McKenna (1995) identified three major assumptions:

- nursing theories lead to better quality of care
- nursing theories have an uncertain effect on quality of care
- nursing theories lower the quality of care.

He undertook an action research approach to implement a nursing theory in a long-stay psychiatric area. The theory concerned was the human needs theory of Minshull et al. (1986) previously selected by a population of ward managers ($n = 95$). Within a broader quasi-experimental design, specific quality-of-care indicators were appraised before and after the implementation of the theory. These dependent variables were also monitored on a control ward and data were collected on both wards at one pre-test and two post-test points. Planned change theory was used as a guiding framework for the implementation of the theory (TFR).

Results showed that on the experimental ward there were statistically significant improvements in care quality, clients' and staffs' perception of ward atmosphere, client satisfaction, staffs' views about nursing theories and client dependency levels. No significant changes were noted in practitioner satisfaction levels or practitioners' perception of clients' behaviour. These findings suggested that when implemented through an action research approach, where practitioners were involved as partners in the change process, a nursing theory has positive influences on quality of client care.

But will such findings be adopted by others and create positive differences to future practice? It is reasonable to suggest that nurses are no different from anyone else and research evidence is not a good enough reason in many instances for changing established behaviour.

In TER, the findings may:

- contribute to establishing the worth of the theory in practice or education
- contribute to the generation of ideas for new theory
- lead to a rejection of an existing theory as a guide for practice or curricula
- lead to an existing theory being adapted or revised within practice or education.

Activity 3: Theory evaluation

You will now know that the evaluation of theory focuses on the impact or effect of that theory on processes and outcomes in practice.

Think specifically about your clinical area and what processes and outcomes you would expect to see improve if a theory is introduced. Examples could include improved patient satisfaction, earlier discharge or improved staff satisfaction.

Outline research approaches that you could use to assess whether the changes in processes and outcomes really happened (e.g. patient satisfaction questionnaire).

Empirical relationship between theory and research

From Chapter 3 you will recall that the philosophers Dickoff and James (1968) identified four levels of theory. In Table 8.2 you will note how Donna Diers (1979) related these to research approaches.

Table 8.2 The relationship between levels of theory and levels of research.

Dickoff and James	Donna Diers
Factor-isolating theory: describes and names concepts	Factor-naming or factor-searching research: describes, names a phenomenon, situation or event in order to gain new insights, called descriptive or exploratory research
Factor-relating theory: relates named concepts to one another	Factor-relating or relation-searching research: develops links among variables and describes the relationships that emanate from factor-searching research – may be qualitative or quantitative
Situation-relating theory: forms interrelationship among concepts or propositions	Explanatory/correlational research aims to determine factors that occur or vary together – no attempt is made to experiment
Situation-producing theory: prescribes actions to reach certain outcomes	Causal hypothesis testing: research addresses causal relationships between variables in an attempt to predict events

Building on this hierarchy of theories it is possible to identify three main types of theory and their related research methods.

Descriptive theory

There are two types of descriptive theory – naming theories and taxonomies (classification theories). Descriptive theories are generated and tested by descriptive research generally called descriptive/exploratory research. The sorts of research questions asked within descriptive studies are: What is this? or: What are the characteristics of . . . ? Descriptive studies involve the observation of phenomena in their natural setting. Data collection can be qualitative (e.g. case studies, ethnography, phenomenology, grounded theory and so on) or quantitative (surveys of attitudes, attributes, knowledge and opinions).

Explanatory theory

This type of theory focuses on relationships between dimensions or characteristics of individuals, groups, situations or events. They explain how the parts of the phenomena under study relate to each other. These theories can only be formulated once phenomena have been identified through descriptive theories having previously been developed. Explanatory theories are developed through explanatory (qualitative) or correlational (quantitative) studies. An example of a research question would be: To what extent is age related to dependency?

Data for explanatory theories may be collected through the use of surveys (observations, interviews, questionnaires) yielding quantitative or qualitative data. Closed-ended instruments may also be used because the parts of the phenomena are believed to be already known as a result of the existence of descriptive theories. To prove a correlation, qualitative data may be transformed into quantitative data and statistical tests such as Pearson product moment coefficient (parametric) or Spearman's Rho (non-parametric) applied. Other more sophisticated tests such as multiple regression and path analysis may also be used.

Predictive theory

This type of theory goes beyond whether one thing is related to another and seeks to identify cause-and-effect relationships. Predictive theories may build on explanatory theories and are generated and tested by experimental research. An example of a question addressed could be: What will happen if you give specific information before surgery? Quantitative data are required to seek statistical significance. Tests include the Mann–Whitney U test (non-parametric) and t-test, ANOVA and MANOVA (parametric).

Therefore, if little is known about the phenomena, descriptive (descriptive theory) research is required. However, if phenomena have been adequately described, correlational (explanatory theory) research may be carried out. If phenomena have been adequately described and relationships are well known then experimental (predictive theory) research may be carried out (see Table 8.3).

Quantitative and qualitative methods are mutually supportive and can provide the researcher with binocular vision of the phenomena under study which neither can provide when used in isolation.

Table 8.3 Relationships between types of theory and research methods.

Theory	Descriptive	Explanatory	Predictive
Research	Qualitative descriptive	Qualitative explanatory	Quantitative experimental
	Quantitative descriptive	Quantitative correlational	

Table 8.4 Carper's ways of knowing as related to research approach (Chinn & Kramer 2004).

Way of knowing	Mode of enquiry
Empirics	Scientific research
Ethics	Dialogue about justice
Personal knowing	Reflection on the congruity between the authentic and disclosed selves
Aesthetics	Critique of the act of nursing

From Chapter 3 readers will recall that Carper (1978) identified four different ways of knowing in nursing. Chinn and Kramer (2004) demonstrate how each is guided by a particular mode of enquiry (Table 8.4).

Strategies for theory development through research

Meleis (2007) identified five major strategies for theory development:

- theory-practice-theory
- practice-theory
- research-theory
- theory-research-theory
- practice-theory-research-theory.

Theory-practice-theory strategy

Here theory from other disciplines is implemented in nursing and becomes shared knowledge. For example, the application from physiology of adaptation theory led to the formulation of Roy's (1980) theory. Similarly, systems theory, when applied in nursing, led to the development of Neuman's (1995) theory.

Practice-theory strategy

The discerning reader will note the relationship of this strategy to TGR. According to Meleis (2007), here theory emanates from clinical experience. The process usually starts when the clinician has a nagging hunch about some phenomena. She develops concepts and describes definitions, boundaries and examples of these concepts. This strategy is based heavily upon Glaser and Strauss's (1967) grounded theory approach where the theorist keeps diaries, observes, analyses similarities and differences, and develops concepts and then linkages. Orlando (1961), Travelbee (1966) and Wiedenbach (1964) used these methods. They became immersed in the clinical area either giving care themselves or observing others doing so. They collected data using case studies, interviews and observations.

Research-theory strategy

This strategy is also related to TGR. This is an inductive approach using four steps (Reynolds 1971: 140):

1 Select a phenomenon that occurs frequently – list all its characteristics.
2 Measure characteristics in a variety of settings.
3 Analyse resultant data to determine systematic patterns worthy of further attention.
4 Formalise these patterns as theoretical statements (axioms).

Proponents of this strategy believe truth exists that can be captured through the senses and verified or refuted. Repeated verification is indicative of truth and prompts the development of scientific theories.

Theory-research-theory strategy

This strategy shows similarities with the TTR approaches outlined above. The following four steps are followed:

1 A theory is selected that explains the phenomena of interest.
2 Concepts of the theory are redefined and operationalised for research.
3 Findings are synthesised and used to modify, refine or develop the original theory.
4 In some instances the result may be a new theory.

Practice-theory-research-theory strategy

There are seven stages in this strategy. These are:

- taking in
- description of phenomenon
- labelling
- concept development
- proposition development
- explicating assumptions
- sharing and communicating.

Meleis (2007) stated that these seven steps may not occur linearly, rather they may occur simultaneously or out of sequence.

Taking in

A clinical situation has attracted a nurse's attention and she develops a hunch about it. She may have observed this event not only through her eyes but through her other senses and through mental activity. The result is 'attention grabbing' which may occur concurrently or retrospectively. The *attention-grabbing* phase is followed by the *attention-giving* phase, a more deliberate process. She may ask the following questions:

- What has attracted my attention?
- Why does it happen?
- Is it similar or different from happenings under different sets of circumstances?
- Under what conditions do I observe it, see it, hear it, touch it?
- Can I describe it?
- Can I document it with theory cases and prototype situations?

Description of phenomenon

At this second stage she should attempt to answer a further set of questions:

- What is the phenomenon?
- When does it occur?
- What are its boundaries?
- Does it vary? Under what circumstances?
- Does it have a function?
- Is it related to time or place?

Another way to begin the description of a phenomenon is by asking questions which start:

- Why do patients . . . ? or
- What is it that happens when . . . ? or
- What are the properties of . . . ?

To ensure that the phenomena are of specific interest to nurses and nursing it is a good idea to attempt answers to some further questions:

- In what way is the phenomenon related to nursing's substantive knowledge base?
- In what way would understanding the phenomenon contribute to understanding some aspect of nursing care?
- Can I think of some questions relating to the phenomenon, the answers to which would be significant to nursing?
- How is the phenomenon related to what nursing policy is?

For instance, a nurse may observe that most of the falls on a ward for older people occur after mealtimes. This is a beginning observation that may evolve into a phenomenon. As similar observations occur the nurse can ask questions of other staff, read and reflect. The end result would be an in-depth description of a phenomenon.

Labelling

In the above example the nurse labels the phenomenon with a word or a short phrase. What she is in essence doing is identifying a concept which best describes the phenomenon. These labels should be concise and precise, used consistently when referring to the phenomenon, contain one cardinal idea and be fundamental to the definition/description of the phenomenon. In the above case the nurse may label the observed phenomenon 'postprandial collapse'.

Concept development

Table 8.5 shows techniques identified by Meleis as appropriate ways of developing concepts.

Proposition development

Propositions may be developed to describe the properties of the concept. This development of propositional statements is a further step in the process of theory development. As outlined earlier, in Table 8.1, there

Table 8.5 Developing concepts (Meleis 2007).

Activity	Rationale
Defining	Here you seek definitions/synonyms of the concept
Differentiating	Here you ask how does this concept differ from similar concepts
Delineating antecedents	Here you define the context and part of this relates to identifying what precedes the occurrence of the concept
Delineating consequences	Here you identify what results from, or follows, the occurrence of the concept. Positive as well as negative consequences should be identified
Modelling	Here cases, contrary and like cases, are identified to help depict what the concept is and what it is not
Analogising	Here the concept is compared with similar concepts which have been studied more extensively. This may help to shed more light on what the new concept is
Synthesising	Here you bring together the findings, meanings and properties that have been amplified by the previous processes

are different types of propositions and the more developed propositions are, the more they are able to define, explain and predict the nature of the relationship between concepts.

Explicating assumptions

The observer reflects on the concepts and propositions and identifies both explicit and implicit assumptions. Reflections on one's own views, values and beliefs will help to delineate assumptions. Assumptions were also dealt with in Chapter 5.

Sharing and communicating

This step goes beyond publishing and presenting at conferences. It involved seminars, conference presentations, journal clubs and other forums where theoretical issues are discussed.

In conclusion, it is important that nurse researchers are aware of the part their study will play in the generation, testing or evaluation of theory. One way of checking this is to answer the following questions (Moody 1990):

- What is the nature and scope of the research aims: exploratory, descriptive, explanatory, predictive?
- Did an existing theory provide the initial idea for the research?
- Is the aim of the study to test existing concepts or propositions from a theory?
- Were study concepts or propositions derived from an existing theory?
- Is the purpose of the study to describe or understand phenomena and from these phenomena develop descriptive or explanatory theory?
- What predominant worldview is reflected in the nature of the research questions?
- Has there been much theoretical progress undertaken on this particular topic?

Slevin (1995) asked us to imagine that theory, practice and research are three dancers. This is a useful metaphor. The dancers interact to produce a systematic and aesthetic beauty and elegance. One weak dancer who stumbles or does not undertake the appropriate movements would cause problems for all three and such a passenger can only be 'carried' for so long. Therefore, all three partners need to be strong and skilled. Similarly, research with weak theory or practice with weak research would be the death knell of nursing as a discipline. It is in our interests to keep these three components strong and ensure that they interact appropriately.

Summary

This chapter gave particular emphasis to the linkages between research and theory. Four links were identified: theory-generating research, theory-testing research, theory-framed research and theory-evaluating research. All four were discussed at length and their contribution to the knowledge base of nursing was explored.

Various authors have also examined the linkages between theory, practice and research (Young et al. 2001). Chinn and Kramer (2004) built on Carper's (1978) work and specified how the four ways of knowing are related to methods of enquiry. Similarly, Donna Diers (1979) constructed a taxonomy of research–theory relationships by building on the work of Dickoff and James (1968). Meleis (2007) identified five distinct strategies highlighting the linkages.

Evaluating Nursing Theories

'This isn't right. It's not even wrong.'

Wolfgang Ernst Pauli (1900–1958)

Outline of content

The importance of establishing 'value' is introduced, including a critique of what we might mean by valuing theory. Terminology that is characteristic of evaluation while at the same time problematic in terms of meaning is explored. The characteristics of a theory are reviewed and expressed in terms of the attributes or dimensions of a 'good' theory. These attributes are presented as the basis for evaluating a theory. The particular place of testing a theory is considered, and the relationship between theory evaluation and theory testing clarified. The usability criterion is presented as an important consideration in nursing, in respect of the theory–practice relationship, and is proposed together with others as a core evaluation criterion.

The famous quotation above, attributed to the physicist Wolfgang Pauli, has been very influential in the philosophy of science as well as in the general scientific literature. Numerous books and papers have been written on the basis of this brief quotation (Burkeman 2005). Some have even taken their title from it. The story runs as follows (see Peierls 1960). One of Pauli's colleagues asked his opinion on a scientific paper.

Pauli's response was (and still is) considered the ultimate scientific putdown: not only was the paper not right in its claims, it was not even wrong! Pauli, a notably biting critic, apparently spoke the words with a sense of sadness and regret. This no doubt made the criticism even more devastating.

But what was Pauli stating here? The first part, that the paper was not right in its claims, seems fairly straightforward: but, what about the second part? What he appeared to be suggesting was that the paper was so vague and imprecise in its claims that you could not even say it was wrong. However, there was more to it than that. To get some idea about this you may wish to review the statements about *refutation* and *falsification* in Chapters 2 and 3. It was claimed there that the 'value' of knowledge (and thus the value of theory as a form of knowledge expression), is established not on the verification of its truth-value or true-ness, but on its openness to refutation or falsification. That is, it is presented in such a way (in sufficiently precise and operational terms) that it *can* be challenged, and as a consequence found to be 'right' or 'wrong'.

This means that as such challenges are repeatedly mounted and defeated, the value of the knowledge is enhanced. Indeed, even if the challenges *are not* repelled, and as a consequence the knowledge (or theory constructed upon it) is found to be unsound, this is also highly valuable: it helps us to establish and carry forward the overall body of knowledge within our discipline, retaining that which has value and discarding that which fails the tests of authenticity. Pauli was therefore suggesting that the paper was so bad that it was not even possible to claim its wrong-ness. We need to know what is wrong every bit as much as we need to know what is right. We will return shortly to the notions of right and wrong.

The importance of this position will perhaps now become clear to you. We have argued earlier in this book that theory can (and should) guide our practice. This is a matter of some magnitude. We are nurses, our interventions – at least sometimes – have the potential to kill or cure. For the remainder of the time, our practices are almost always highly important. For the ill person, even the way a glass of water is presented, or the manner in which a need to void is being met, become issues of magnitude. We *need* to know something about whether (using Pauli's terminology) the theory guiding this practice is right or at least not wrong.

You will have noted we are confronted with these terms *right* and *wrong* again. It must be acknowledged that we cannot expect or indeed depend upon absolutes here. We will *never* have absolute truth; there *is* no unequivocal and unassailable right or wrong. The best theories are no more than those that have repeatedly withstood challenges sufficiently that we can with a high degree of confidence prescribe our interventions on their basis. If we do not know that the information or knowledge or theory is right (or at least right for now, on the basis of the evidence and reasoning that is at our disposal), and if it is so imprecisely or imperfectly stated that it is impossible to challenge it or show it to be wrong, it is useless to us (at least in respect of guiding practice). We have not even got to the point of addressing in a constructive manner what we might mean by evaluation, and what evaluating the worth of a theory may entail. However, we can anticipate that the need for theory to be clearly stated so that it can be challenged (and thereby strengthened or refuted) perhaps identifies the first two issues that are important in evaluating theory, outlined in Table 9.1.

So, what have we established in these opening comments? We confirm once again, as we have throughout this book, that theory is vitally important to nursing. We *do* need a body of knowledge to inform and guide our practice. We need to be sure that it is sound, or dependable, or right. This latter sentence points us to two issues: we need to know the value of the theory; but the way we express this value is highly problematic as we have to resort to terms such as 'sound', 'dependable' and 'right'.

Even in Table 9.1, and the subsequent tables that extend this listing as the chapter progresses, we are using terms such as 'good' and 'worthy'. This is fine: it *does* help convey our general meanings. But be aware that the terms are problematic. Just as there are problems with terms such as 'right' and 'wrong', there are difficulties with words such as 'good' and 'worthy'. Let us for now assume the term *good* means (in the context intended here) an acceptable standard or quality, of value to the nursing purpose in the sense that it has a goodness of fit. Insofar as it meets this fitness for purpose the theory is worthy or commendable as useful to nursing.

In the remainder of the chapter, we consider the difficulties of terminology, the nature of value and evaluation, and the processes and procedures we might employ in evaluating theory. We start with the terminology. It may seem to the reader that it is pedestrian to be constantly questioning the terminology. However, it is only by adopting this critical stance that we can arrive at a position whereby we can really form reasoned and balanced views on a theory's worth.

Table 9.1 The evaluation dimensions I.

A good or worthy theory will: 1 be expressed in precise, clear and operational terms that allow us to test it *(Parsimony and Testability)* 2 withstand challenges to refute or falsify it, while being open to or facilitating such challenges *(Defeasibility)*

Activity 1: Science and knowledge

We will be concerned with how within science knowledge is constructed into theory, which is then tested and evaluated. It may be helpful to review and reflect upon the nature of ideas and how we use them to construct knowledge.

Listen to the interview of and talk by Professor Peter Godfrey-Smith of Harvard University. This can be found as a free podcast download on the iTunes internet website, under the 'iTunes U' section within the iTunes online store (the section devoted to higher/university education). You do not need any particular brand of MP3 player to use the iTunes podcasts, but you *do* need to have the iTunes application on your Windows PC or Apple Macintosh computer. You can download the podcast, listen to it on your PC or Mac, download it to your MP3 player and listen to it there, or burn it from iTunes onto a CD-ROM disk and listen to it from any CD music player or PC.

The podcast can also be sourced as follows:

1   Go to Stanford University website. The URL is http://itunes.stanford.edu
2   The website will redirect you automatically to the iTunes online store and its iTunes U section for Stanford University. If the website does not function, you can still access the podcast free by directly accessing the iTunes online store (see above).
3   Follow the path thus: open 'Arts and Humanities', then open 'Philosophy', then open 'Philosophy of Science' (this is the Godfrey-Smith podcast). Download should occur automatically.

Listen to the podcast – it lasts around 1 hour. Take notes as you listen, particularly in respect of the discussions on how ideas make contact with experience to lead to the construction of knowledge. You may wish to follow this up by returning to Chapter 3 and noting the major points on knowledge in that chapter.

Reflect on the fact that in this chapter you will be considering not the evaluation of policies or programmes, but the evaluation of ideas as constructed into theory, and the further impact of these artefacts (ideas, knowledge, theory) upon practice.

The support of Apple Inc, The Apple Store and Stanford University are acknowledged in making freely available to all students and the academic community the resources on iTunes U

The words that pave our path

Right and wrong

You will have noted the sense of reservation creeping in with respect to how certain words are used. This relates particularly to the words *right* and *wrong*. It may also be important in respect of other terms. We do fully appreciate that this constant re-examining of words may at times be highly irritating to you, as you move through the book. But it is necessary to do this, in order that we arrive at workable ways forward. Let us take these first two words (right and wrong), and consider how they may be used.

1 *Absolute truth*: By *right*, we may mean that a piece of factual or cognitive knowledge, or perhaps even a whole theory constructed from it, is accurate. That is, it is absolutely and irrevocably true – it fully and accurately reflects some aspect of our external (or perhaps even internal) world. By contrast, *wrong* implies the complete opposite: the knowledge is false, or wrong, or inaccurate, or unsound – and it is totally so.

2 *Truth as relative and contextual*: A similar but less dogmatic position may see these expressions of *right* and *wrong* as being essentially expressions of goodness of fit. The claims to truth (or falsehood) are based upon the extent that they have a degree of evidence or reason on their side. This is further supported by the way in which that which is considered *right* is seen to have fitness for purpose: it makes sense within the social or cultural context, and while it may not make sense elsewhere, here it can be seen to serve a useful purpose. In this sense of the two terms, people *do* recognise the dangers of making extreme claims about what is true or false. It *is* recognised that new information sometimes comes along to completely change how we see things. Therefore, when people use the terms right and wrong here, they are recognising that they are *conditional* terms: they are right and wrong, in these circumstances, at this particular time.

3 *Moral contexts of rightness and wrongness*: Of course, both the above positions are about right and wrong as factual matters. There is a sense in which the terms *right* and *wrong* instead refer to moral matters. It is *right* to do some things, to think in certain ways; it is *wrong* to do other things, to think in other ways. Here, we are using the terms as ethical constructs. Something may be adjudged to be *morally* right, in so far as it is morally *good* and is expressed as a *virtue*. Conversely, something may be adjudged *morally* wrong, in so far as it is morally *bad* and is expressed as a *vice*.

This linking of right with virtuousness and wrong with viciousness has little to do with propositional knowledge or theory constructed from this, although it is of course an area of vital importance in nursing. Indeed, some would argue that propositional knowledge construction is not relevant in respect of rightness in this ethical sense. According to this argument, we do not need any complex reasoning, or any empirical evidence, to confirm that killing or incest is *wrong*, or that showing mercy and compassion is *right*. They are taken as self-evident characteristics of human virtue. It may be recalled that in Chapter 2 it was suggested that it is this moral dimension rather than our capacity to reason that defines our humanness.

There are ethical positions that do not conform to the latter thinking. In contrast to the latter position, sometimes termed the deontological position (that right is based upon universal principles that are self-evident, and is right irrespective of consequences), there is a teleological position (that right is based upon the outcomes of our thoughts and actions, and depends on the causes or consequences of our actions insofar as these outcomes may be good or beneficial to ourselves and/or others). In the latter instance, a common position is that of 'the greatest good' principle. This suggests that what is right or good morally is that which conveys the most advantages – or 'goodness' – to the greatest number of people. Here it can be seen that propositional thinking and reason *is* involved, at least in terms of working out net advantages. This is beyond our main remit in this chapter. Suffice it to say that our main concerns here are with the first two meanings of right and wrong. However, we briefly return to this issue of a moral dimension later, when we consider the different attributes of a theory that must be addressed in evaluation.

Evaluation and worth

Worth is an expression of value – when we ask what something is worth, we are asking about its value. The process or method by which we arrive at a statement of worth or value is termed *evaluation*. The term seems fairly straightforward. It is arriving at a statement of *value* or *worth* in respect of the phenomenon under examination. The term 'evaluation and worth' seems to be something of a tautology – a meaningless repetition of words. It is almost as if we are asking about placing value (worth) on the worth (value) of something: what is the value of the value! But this is not as meaningless as it seems. The issue of value may be straightforward (at least to some extent) if that which we are valuing can be measured. Here, we can establish the value of something by stating its value or worth in concrete terms. If one automobile tyre lasts for 15,000 miles before its treads begin to disappear and another lasts for 30,000 miles before the same degree of wear appears, we can formulate a standard. If each 150 miles of travel costs 50 pence of tyre use we can say the first tyre is worth £50 while the second is worth £100. Of course, the question is: how did we arrive at 150 miles of tyre travel being worth 50 pence in the first place? This is not so much a matter of objective judgement based upon some scientific measure, but the result of complex social and economic influences. Furthermore, if someone can produce a tyre of the same quality as the £100 tyre, or even better, for £80 so that we are paying 40 pence or less for each 150 miles of tyre travel, we feel we have something of better quality. But we also say this is good value – we are getting it at *better* than the going rate, paying less than what is considered the fair exchange across the market.

The value we place on something in terms of the 'worth' we attribute to it is a social construct. It only has a 'worth' because we value it, and this is largely a function of our culture, the social groups we belong to, and so on. It is therefore important, when we come to evaluate theory, to remember that what is being valued is often linked to positions held by specific social groups. Some groups have a vested interest in ensuring that particular outcomes will be achieved. They therefore only want these outcomes to be evaluated and they want them to be evaluated in objective and measurable terms. This might suit a health service manager who wants to demonstrate that evidence (contained in theory) is informing practice (and therefore showing that he is meeting his commitment in respect of clinical governance requirements – his responsibility for clinical standards). Such information may not necessarily be what is needed (or at least not *all* of what is needed) by nurses also interested in the loneliness and isolation experienced by patients with cancer who are receiving chemotherapy.

From Chapter 3 you will recall Galileo's call for everything to be measurable. As we stated there, the problem is that not everything can be measured in objective terms. For example, how might we measure the worth of something like the value attributed to 'being listened to'? Often we hear patients say that 'nobody listened to me, they did not really want to hear my concerns'. This phenomenon (the need to be listened to, to be understood) is clearly highly valued by patients within healthcare systems. But how do we attribute some *worth* to it? We may measure some things around the phenomenon: how often nurses or other healthcare professionals *appear* to be listening to their patients; how patients *seem* to be appreciating this (perhaps using a 5-point measurement scale). But these do not actually measure the values gained by the patient, such as: feelings of appreciation; experiencing reassurance that one is being understood, or that there is at least a genuine attempt to understand; a sense of personhood – of being respected as an individual and of being valued by the listener. We may very well observe a nurse *appearing* to be listening. But are we sure that active listening is occurring and that this nurse is *really* opening herself to the voice of the other? Similarly, we may well ask patients to score their level of appreciation of being listened to. But how do we – and they – differentiate in any real objective sense between a score of 3 and of 4?

Standards and quality

The latter observations draw our attention to the relationship that may exist between standards and quality. When we judge or value something, when we in effect attribute some *worth* to it, we tend to adopt either subjective or objective positions. These depend on a number of influences, but the main ones are the nature of the thing itself, and the orientation of the evaluator. Some things can, to a greater or lesser extent, be measured, while others cannot. For instance, the issue of *being listened to* is an example of something that would be very hard (if not impossible) to measure. Other things might be different. For example, the importance of ensuring that patients receive the correct medication is something we value. The quality level or value we aspire to is accurate and safe administration of medicines. It is also something we can measure: by observing and recording we can (leaving aside for the moment difficulties of observing and recording) establish the number of occasions the correct medicine was given to the correct patients, the number of occasions incorrect dosages were given, and so on.

Generally speaking, things we value or aspire to that can also be measured are defined as standards. This raises a question about the relationship between quality and standards. If standards are quantitative measurements, how can they be assumed to be quality statements? Usually, what we are saying here is that these quantitative measures are *indirect indicators* of quality. The standards for correctness and accuracy of medicine administration (as expressed in standards – such as: 'Each patient receives the correct medicine in the correct dosage') are not a direct measure of a quality we might label as 'safety'. But they *do* give an indirect measure that suggests or makes it reasonable to assume that the quality we term safety is being met.

A problem does exist, however, where there is a tendency to attempt to measure everything. This is why we suggest above that the orientation of the evaluator is important. Sometimes, those attempting to establish quality adopt a perspective that seems to assume that everything associated with quality *can* be measured. However, some aspects of quality are not capable of measurement in this sense, and even those things that *are* measures of quality are not actually measuring quality directly but are measuring things that – we claim – indirectly signify quality.

All this leaves us with a question: if we cannot directly *measure* quality, how do we demonstrate its presence? Our arguments above can be summarised to answer this question as follows: Quality is expressed through:

- *standards* – objective measures which point indirectly to the presence of quality;
- *descriptors* – non-objective statements which endeavour to express the nature of quality in a given situation.

If we accept the above statements, we might see something like the following emerging:

Within the hospital, there is an ethos of learning and inquiry. This emphasises the importance of lifelong learning as part of the means of achieving and maintaining best clinical practices. (Descriptor)

Each member of staff has an agreed development action plan that guarantees a minimum of five study days per annum. (Standard)

When we use a term like descriptor, and use it to identify terms such as an ethos, we are often open to criticism. The term, taken from the ancient Greek *ethos* meaning character, can have a wide range of meanings. It can relate to a place, an organisation, a person, a group of people. It concerns the nature of that place or those people, their disposition or attitude or outlook, their culture and what they value within it. It has something in the nature of an ambience to it – an atmosphere or feel. But it goes beyond this. It is a fundamental way of being that is so much an essential part of the place or the organisation or the group that it is experienced as a powerful presence.

Thus, in the example above, a learning and growing attitude or outlook pervaded the organisation. This term *pervaded* is important; it denotes that the character or characteristic is spread out within, is in fact a part of the place, organisation, person. In a sense, it is its spirit. This is a bit like the idea of tacit knowledge we addressed in Chapters 2 and 3: we 'know' the ethos in the sense that we can feel it or sense it, but we cannot actually *point to it*, we can only point to its *indicators*. It is exactly *because* it is not a concrete entity, because we cannot measure it, that we are open to criticism. Yet most people of insight will know what is being discussed.

In an Accident and Emergency Department, we may see a standard which states 'All patients referred to a doctor will see one within 90 minutes'. People will recognise that while seriously injured or seriously ill people will be seen by a triage nurse on arrival and referred to a doctor almost immediately, there is nevertheless a standard that *everyone* will be seen within 90 minutes. But the ethos that pervades this Accident and Emergency Department, the way people are treated as persons, the palpable feeling that the staff care, is also important. And it is amazing how people sense this. Yet it continues to be problematic just because it *is* imprecise and not describable in concrete, measurable terms.

Furthermore, it is important to remember that the terms we use are sometimes applied loosely and differently. This is not the first time we have encountered such problems. Sometimes people use the term *descriptor* to indicate measurable criteria, and sometimes the term *standard* is used to indicate levels to be aimed for rather than a measure of what is actually achieved. In effect, the descriptor becomes the measurable and the standard the immeasurable! The important point to remember is that quality and quantity are two different things, that they are indeed opposites. One (quality) is immeasurable and identifies the essential characteristics of something; the other (quantity) is measurable and indicates how specific calculable criteria are being met.

Activity 2: Standards and quality

We have recognised that standards are objective, measurable criteria that serve as quality indicators. We have also recognised that some indicators of quality cannot be expressed objectively in measurable terms. We have used the term 'descriptor' to identify these alternatives, because they can only be expressed in descriptive and sometimes only in subjective terms.

A   Consider your areas of healthcare, and in particular the clinical nursing aspect within it.
  1   Write three standards for nursing care (i.e. quality indicators that involve or allow measurement). Clearly state the standard and the measures aimed for in each instance.
  2   Write three descriptors for nursing care (i.e. quality indicators that cannot be stated objectively in measurable terms). Ensure that, while measurement is not possible, the descriptor is written in clear and precise terms.
  3   Consider how these statements might contribute to evaluating the quality of nursing interventions.

B   Theories are mostly expressed in measurable terms. We have
     noted earlier that the characteristics of middle range theory and
     practice theory are that they are expressed in operational terms
     that can be observed and (mostly) measured. Research that
     tests such theory is usually quantitative. However, other
     research is of a more qualitative nature and it does not produce
     theory in the same way – or at least theory in a testable form.
     1   Briefly explore the literature on qualitative research, iden-
          tifying the product or outcomes obtained from such
          research.
     2   Obtain from this literature a brief outline of how such
          research is evaluated, including how its impact upon prac-
          tice is evaluated.

Quality as essence

The whole idea of quality as a term that denotes something that is
immeasurable – cannot be directly observed, cannot be measured in
quantitative terms – is problematic. It places *quality* alongside such
notions as love, spirituality, soul, and even those aspects of goodness
we discussed earlier that were termed ethical or moral. Indeed, the
concept of *ethos* that we alluded to above is another such example. Such
things have a nature or essence that is difficult to define. They are by
definition beyond measurement, yet can be powerfully recognised.

We can get into a certain Eastern European car and we sense the
tackiness even before we see that there are measurable deficits (poor
build standards). When we sit in a Rolls Royce we can of course see
the very high build standards that are measurable. But there is something else there also. There is a whole sense of the value of the thing –
its looks, its feel, even its smell tells us we are in the presence of
something that is special and essentially superior. It is a bit like the
earlier example of a good Accident and Emergency Department: there
are of course all the measurable standards, but there is also this sense
in which it exudes quality (and we used the term ethos to refer to this
earlier).

We can see this in almost everything around us. You all know that
you can go to a certain high street store and buy a pair of jeans for £10,
and that you can go elsewhere and buy a pair for £100. People may say
you are crazy to pay ten times the price for what is nothing more than
a pair of trousers made out of denim. But *you* know, of course, that
there is a cut to these trousers, a feel to the denim, an experience of
how they 'sit' or 'hang' that exudes something, and we term this something quality. Of course your critics will say that you are hoodwinking

yourself, that fools are easily parted from their money. But more often than not your *experiencing* of quality in this item is borne out: three years later these jeans still feel great on you, they still retain their shape and style. In that time you may have got by with only buying six pairs of the £10 jeans! You could have saved £40! But, would you have spent three years in shapeless mediocrity, and would it have been worth £40?

Of course, sometimes we *are* fools who are being easily parted from our money. We may think, just because something costs £100 rather than £10, just because it has a certain brand name, it is by definition high quality. This is not always the case. However, we can usually tell (although some *are* better at this than others) when we are in the presence of quality.

Note again the above phrase: 'in the presence of quality'. The author Robert Pirsig (1974, 1993) suggested that quality was indeed an essential or natural state that could be aspired to. Things in themselves do not, he argued, define or establish quality. Quality is an essence (like air, or human kindness) that things can be open to, can embrace, or alternatively turn away from. We can sometimes sense this in theory also. It has about it an ambience that is illuminating and meaning-unfolding. Such theory is often expressed in terms so simple and so parsimonious that its insight-producing power bursts upon us. We know immediately how it illuminates, how it explains, almost without any need to submit it to tests. It contains within it such a simplicity of 'rightness' that we do not understand how *we ourselves* did not see it all along. Einstein's $e = mc^2$ representing the theory of relativity has an elegance about it. Also, when Watson and Crick worked out the structure of DNA they remarked how beautiful it looked.

Value and theory

In this section we have considered some of the terms that are associated with evaluation. The four issues we addressed were:

- right and wrong
- evaluation and worth
- standards and quality
- quality as essence

Right and wrong

In evaluating theory, we will be concerned with whether the knowledge contained within the theory is accurate, or the *best available knowledge* under the circumstances, even though we accept that absolute truth or rightness is not a useful concept. We will furthermore expect this knowledge – as it is theoretical – to *describe, explain or even predict* in respect of the phenomena it addresses.

Evaluation and worth

We will also be concerned with how we value the theory (and the knowledge contained within it). We might of course value something that approximates truth or rightness, for its own sake. But in nursing, the *worth* of the theory will be associated with its usefulness: the theory will be required to have *utility*. Assuming the knowledge is adjudged to be sound, and has consistently withstood the attempts at falsification we referred to earlier, we might furthermore expect it to have *prescriptive* power.

Standards and quality

While we appreciate that there is a difference between standards (insofar as these are defined as quantifiable, measurable conditions) and quality that is largely unquantifiable (by definition it is quality, not quantity), we nevertheless recognise how *standards are useful indicators* of quality, while quality descriptors help us centre upon what is being valued.

Quality as essence

Finally, we might perhaps recognise that quality is an essential phenomenon that is sensed and to which we can open ourselves and what we do – including the doing or formulation of nursing theories.

By considering these terms and the difficulties they present to us, we are more readily prepared to proceed to the more specific consideration of theory evaluation. But we have also, in carrying this discussion forward, proceeded to present further criteria for evaluating a theory. Drawing upon the above four issues, we can add to the dimensions of a good or worthy theory presented previously in Table 9.1. The six additional dimensions (drawn from the above four issues) are presented as items 3–8 in Table 9.2.

Of course, we will be returning to the processes of theory evaluation in more detail below. But it can be seen that in addressing these important wider considerations we have progressed some way along this road.

Table 9.2 The evaluation dimensions II.

A good or worthy theory will:
1   be expressed in precise, clear and operational terms that allow us to test it
    (Parsimony and Testability)
2   withstand challenges to refute or falsify it, while being open to or facilitating
    such challenges (Defeasibility)
3   present, on the basis of the latter, the best available knowledge on the
    particular topic at the particular time (Evidence and Justified True Belief)
4   organise and express this knowledge in such a way that it (the theory)
    describes, and/or explains, and/or predicts phenomena and the relationships
    or links between them (Coherence and Consistency)
5   be useful or have utility in the practice of nursing (Utility)
6   where it (the theory) does have utility for nursing, furthermore have withstood
    the challenges to its predictive powers consistently to the point where there is
    confidence in utilising it to prescribe nursing actions (Prescriptive Value)
7   identify or underpin certain standards and descriptors that pertain to quality
    of nursing care (Quality Enhancement)
8   contain within it an essential nature that conveys its value as a source of
    nursing insight, a sense in which it illuminates nursing or a part of the nursing
    world (Meaningfulness)

Testing and evaluating theory

Differentiation

It is important to make a distinction between testing and evaluating theory. This is not always easy. As we have discovered throughout this book, people tend to use words differently and not always with complete clarity. Therefore, the distinction we make here is provisional, and we acknowledge that there is not universal agreement.

To ease our way through this matter, the distinction we are proceeding to make is as follows:

* *Testing* is an initial process in the life of a theory, whereby untested theory is being tested through the research process.
* *Evaluation* is a process concerned with establishing the value, or worth, or utility of a theory that has usually been already tested through research and is now being applied or used in practice.

Testing

The idea that we test theory by a process of research depends to some extent on acceptance of the premise that theory is linked with scientific endeavour. As we discovered earlier in this book, this is not universally accepted. Nevertheless, prominent figures in science, including Popper (1989) and Kuhn (1962) have argued that theory is a vitally important aspect in the successful progression of a discipline and in the establishment of a reliable body of knowledge. It has of course been argued that theory has also the capacity to influence how we see reality. As David Bohm (1998a) suggested, a theory is a lens through which we view the world. Such lenses help us to make sense of this world. But as Bohm pointed out, the lens of one theory (indeed of one discipline) may be very different to that of another. Indeed, Popper (1994) expressed concern about how opposing theories may be so firmly entrenched and so opposed that there is no openness to dialogue among their proponents. Here Popper departs from, and indeed is highly critical of, the view of Kuhn (1962) that paradigms and their expanding bodies of knowledge are positive and even essential aspects of science. He suggested that these worldviews might in fact tie us into particular outlooks and essentially block open dialogue across paradigms that might enhance understanding. Even in his book title *The Myth of the Framework* Popper (1994) expresses his cutting criticism of imposed and blinkered worldviews.

As long as we recognise the limitations of a theory, we can proceed to maximise its usefulness in our day-to-day lives. But before we get to this point, let us return just for a moment to the ideas of tested and untested theories. And let us refresh our memories: theory plus research (one argument holds) are together the components of science. Theory is taken as the creative process by which we postulate descriptions, explanations, or predictions about how things are in the world. Such *postulated theories* are by definition *untested theories*. Research is taken as the practical or empirical procedures by which we then test the theories, under strictly controlled laboratory conditions. Where this is not possible or it is adjudged inappropriate (for example, in some aspects of the social and human sciences that require study in their natural settings), we test the theory in real-world conditions under the best controls available (using rigorous research methods). Theories that 'pass' the test(s) are termed *tested theory*. In the philosophy of science, the traditional test for knowledge is known as the establishment of *justified true belief*. This is a concept we discussed in some detail in Chapter 2. Using that terminology here, in theory testing we seek evidence to *justify* our *belief* in the theory's claims in respect of what is being held to be *true*.

There are two additional points we should remind ourselves about here.

- As we noted earlier (Chapters 2 and 3) science has moved from rigid positivistic positions characterised by quests for absolute truths and knowledge that is irrevocably true and correct, to a post-positivistic era. In this newer era, wherein it is recognised that absolute truth and knowledge that is irrevocably and permanently accurate is an impossible quest, we instead adjudge knowledge (or theory) by the extent to which it is constantly and consistently refuted through challenges or attempts to falsify (i.e. demonstrate its unsoundness). Therefore, tested theory is only taken as the best theory for now, and always the very next challenge may refute it. In essence, theory must always be under test; there is no permanent and reliable *state* that we may term tested theory and it is always the best we have for now.

- When we proceed to the issue of evaluation later, we shall largely be concerned with the aforementioned *tested* theory. However, it is important that this does not lead us to the conclusion that untested theory is in some sense inferior. Indeed, it is the gift of imagination and insight that leads to creative theory postulation and marks the divide between mundane number crunching and scientific excellence. It might well seem, when we in nursing are at the 'end-user' point, i.e. of using theory in practice, that the really important factor is tested theory that has emerged from high quality research, particularly where the research presents evidence that supports the predictive powers of tested theory so that we can utilise it to guide practice. We spoke of this in Chapter 2 as *prescriptive theory*.

However, way back before all of this, before the application of the tested theory, before its testing in research, and before the untested theory was expressed in a theory format, there was the creative thinking that led to the original formulation of the theory. Someone was original enough in their thinking, insightful enough in their reflections, and courageous enough in their openness to what the world out there was conveying to them to say, 'Ah, this is how it might be!'

Activity 3: Any monkey can do research

The above title is meant to be provocative. It is of course the case that in some forms of research fairly mundane questions are constructed and a questionnaire is administered. Then the researcher enters the data into a statistical package and presents the findings in a report that is largely of a proforma type: frequencies are presented and sometimes colourful pie charts and bar graphics are used to illustrate findings. The literature reporting such research is replete with phrases such as 'It has been found that there is an association between eating milk chocolate and acne in adolescents.'

It is perhaps an exaggeration to suggest that monkeys might be trained to conduct such research, although it is possible that they might indeed be trained to conduct parts of such processes more effectively than humans! But what is really being suggested here is that the creative thinking part of science, the formulations of possible explanations, the making of predictions that can then be tested, is what really makes the difference between mundane fact finding and excellent science.

David Bohm has said: 'there are a tremendous number of highly talented people who remain mediocre'. Thus, there must have been a considerable body of scientists who were better at mathematics and knew more physics than Einstein did. The difference was that Einstein had 'a certain quality of originality' (Bohm 1998b: 3). It was this originality, and the capacity to become immersed in the subject, to seek new ways of unfolding the meaning that was enfolded within things, that according to Bohm characterises the creative thinker.

Reflect upon the importance of creative thinking in theorising. Look up terms that relate to this issue, including creativity, originality, imagination and innovation. Write a 250-word statement that defines or explains the essential characteristics of creativity.

Do you feel creativity as you have defined it is an important attribute of theory and theorising?

As we noted earlier, sometimes people use the various terms (testing, assessing, appraising, evaluating, and so on) interchangeably. However, we take the view that *theory testing* is a more precise term, concerned specifically with the researching of a theory. That is, as suggested above, once a theory is originally postulated, it must then be tested through research. However, we should not assume that this is a static thing. As demonstrated in Figure 9.1, there is a cyclical process at play. Even after a theory is tested through research, when it is used in the real-world situation over time, it may emerge that there are some aspects that lack a goodness of fit. This may (as indicated in Figure 9.1) lead to further theorising, the outcome of which is a further untested theory. This in turn must then be tested, and so the process proceeds in a cyclical fashion.

This is of course something of a simplification. It might be taken from Figure 9.1 that the only source of untested theory is the use of theory in practice. This is not necessarily the case, as would be suggested by our earlier recognition of the importance of original thinking in creative science. Similarly, our practice may be informed by sources other than tested theory, as may be recalled when we discussed atheoretical *know-how* practical knowledge in Chapters 2 and 3.

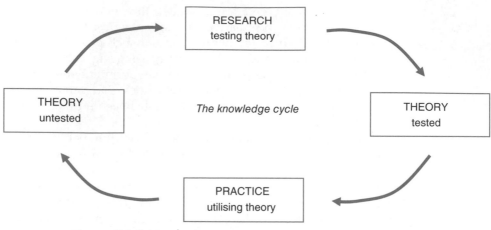

Figure 9.1 Testing theory.

Nevertheless, practice is a rich ground for the further refinement of theory. It is indeed important as it submits the theory to a further test of what we might term *relevance*. Indeed, earlier in this book we considered the approach known as *grounded theory* (Glaser & Strauss 1967) wherein theory is derived from data within the practice situation, so that relevance is by definition an element within all grounded theories.

Evaluating

Thus far we have put forward the position that testing is primarily to do with research, while evaluation is to do with establishing the value or worth of a tested theory. This is illustrated in Figure 9.2. It is important to note that this is also something of a simplification. It is recognised that evaluation is concerned with the effectiveness of tested theory. However, this does not mean that there is only a limited linkage between testing and that which we are terming evaluation. First, evaluation is also a dynamic process: there is a concern not only with how the theory 'performs' in the real-life situation, but also with establishing that it has been effectively tested, using appropriate research methodologies. Second, there is an increasing expectation that evaluation itself will be research based. This is a matter we shall return to presently.

In a sense, theory evaluation is always about evaluating a moving target, it is a dynamic and ongoing process. Theory that is 'good' or

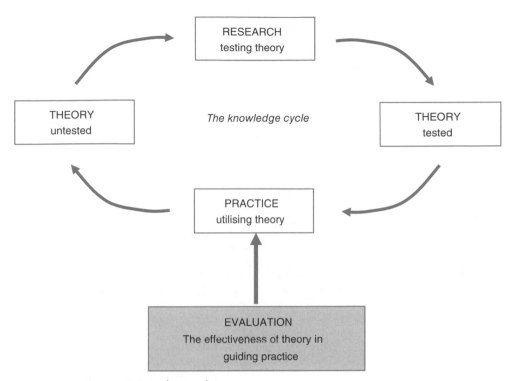

Figure 9.2 Evaluating theory.

that we might to some degree depend upon is established upon a continuing process of being challenged for falsification. How it performs in practice may (as shown in Figure 9.2) lead to further information, and then further testing, and on the basis of this, further reframing of the theory. Furthermore, in seeking to establish the value of a theory, we also address its structural and process dimensions, which may also be constantly changing. That is, the theory as it develops and is refined by research testing and real-world application does not stay static but constantly enhances our insight into the world and its workings. The essence of a good theory is how it unfolds meaning and enhances insight – not just restating current knowledge but presenting new knowledge in an original sense, and/or representing current knowledge in new and creative ways that provide us with new insights. Taking these further dimensions of dynamic refinement and originality, we can add two additional dimensions to our developing view of the dimensions upon which theory can be evaluated, as items 9 and 10 in Table 9.3. Furthermore, in recognition of our above discussion on relevance, we can extend our fifth dimension to incorporate 'relevance and utility'.

Table 9.3 The evaluation dimensions III.

A good or worthy theory will:
1 be expressed in precise, clear and operational terms that allow us to test it *(Parsimony and Testability)*
2 withstand challenges to refute or falsify it, while being open to or facilitating such challenges *(Defeasibility)*
3 present, on the basis of the latter, the best available knowledge on the particular topic at the particular time *(Evidence and Justified True Belief)*
4 organise and express this knowledge in such a way that it (the theory) describes, and/or explains, and/or predicts phenomena and the relationships or links between them *(Coherence and Consistency)*
5 be useful or have utility in the practice of nursing *(Relevance and Utility)*
6 where it (the theory) *does* have utility for nursing, furthermore have withstood the challenges to its predictive powers consistently to the point where there is confidence in utilising it to *prescribe* nursing actions *(Prescriptive Value)*
7 identify or underpin certain standards and descriptors that pertain to quality of nursing care *(Quality Enhancement)*
8 contain within it a sense or essential nature that conveys its value as a source of nursing insight, a sense in which it illuminates nursing or a part of the nursing world *(Meaningfulness)*
9 be established upon a dynamic orientation that assumes testing as an *ongoing* commitment *(Dynamism)*
10 reflects a creative unfoldment that provides new and original meaning as opposed to simply restating current knowledge *(Originality)*

Evaluation as research, theory as focus

There is one final sense in which the activities of testing and evaluation are linked. Within health services, and particularly within the UKs National Health Service, there is an increasing emphasis upon what was originally termed *evidence-based medicine* (EBM) (Sackett et al. 2000) but has been extended to include other disciplines, e.g. evidence-based nursing or evidence-informed nursing (Ingersoll 2000; McSherry et al. 2002). Taking a wider than professional discipline position, vocabulary such as evidence-based practice (irrespective of the professional discipline) or evidence-based health (a term often intended to indicate a comprehensive approach) have become popular variations in the terminology. It is now even recognised that the patient or client who nowadays participate much more fully in their treatment and care must be provided with adequate information to do so – thus leading to the EBM offshoot, evidence-informed patient choice (Entwhistle et al. 1998).

The importance of basing practices on the best available evidence has now extended well beyond medicine and health. It is now recognised that policy and programme management issues must also draw upon the best available evidence. There is therefore a push towards such approaches; the term utilised in the UK is evidence-based policy and practice. This is promoted from government level (Cabinet Office 1999, 2001) and increasingly recognised in the wider academic, research and service delivery communities (Davies et al. 2000; OECD 2001; Pawson 2001, 2002).

It must be recognised that evaluation as an activity often falls within the latter broad remit (of strategy and development, planning, and policy and practice). Insofar as evidence to underpin what we do has become paramount, the establishment of research orientations to procure such evidence also becomes an imperative. Therefore, we find that increasingly strategy and policy is expected to draw on knowledge derived from research. Similarly, when policy and programmes are being evaluated, it is expected that the same rigorous methods as used for other areas of scientific inquiry will apply. According to Weiss:

> 'Doing evaluation through a process of research takes more time and costs more money than offhand evaluations that rely on intuition, opinion, or trained sensibility, but it provides a rigor that is missing in these more informal activities. Rigor is apt to be particularly important when (a) the outcomes to be evaluated are complex, hard to observe, made up of many elements interacting in diverse ways; (b) the decisions that will follow are important and expensive; and (c) evidence is needed to convince other people about the validity of the conclusions.' (Weiss 1998: 5)

A research orientation in evaluation is not a new thing. Within academic circles, evaluative research has a history extending back to the 1930s and beyond. However, as late as the 1970s it was perhaps viewed as one of the softer academic activities (Weiss 1972, 1998). People were not fully decided on the nature of evaluative research (or even upon its title – terms such as *evaluation research* or *outcomes studies* were also being used), or indeed the activities or methods it involved. There were in fact two broad divides in existence:

- First, there was a gap between the idea that evaluation research was a particular form of inquiry with its own methods, and the opposing view that the only specific aspect was the focus of the research (i.e. evaluation) with the research methods being the same as for any other form of research (Childers 1989).
- Second, it was often the case that there was a wide gap between evaluation research and evaluation (without a link to research in its title *or* its orientation). The latter activity was by far the most common, at least up until recent times. Such 'non-research' evaluation largely involved approaches which to a greater or lesser extent

rested upon professional judgement or expert opinion rather than any systematic research activity (Weiss 1972, 1998). The emphasis was very much upon the capacity to bring logical reasoning and experience together in recognising the value of what was being achieved in programmes. Indeed, those involved would often not even have been versed or experienced in research and scientific methods.

Some of what is presented in nursing literature on theory evaluation demonstrates an awareness of the scientific orientation, but is nevertheless a form of evaluation that does not incorporate an empirical dimension. It therefore falls into the second of the above categories, albeit exclusively evaluating from a logical-reasoning viewpoint that excludes experience or personal expertise of the evaluator. This draws to a large extent upon analytic argument and critical appraisal based upon principles of logic, much in line with traditional philosophical as opposed to empirical or scientific modes of inquiry. Indeed, such activities are often identified as being concerns within the realm of what has become known as *nursing philosophy*.

We may very easily find ourselves drawn into another round of controversial argument and counter-argument here, this time about whether there is or can be a nursing philosophy, and if so, what its legitimate areas of activity might be. Suffice for now is to state that there is within nursing a recognition that some areas of nursing can be informed by drawing from the areas of philosophical inquiry. These areas of inquiry include approaches that are epistemological and logical (i.e. concerned with knowledge and its construction), ethical (i.e. concerned with moral issues) or metaphysical (i.e. concerned with the nature of existence of things or beings in the world). The evaluation or critique of theory clearly falls within the first of these three approaches, that is, the area concerned with knowledge and its structure and nature, construction, validity and so on which is named *epistemology* (a term derived from the Greek that translates as 'the study of knowledge').

An inquiry into theory (including the evaluation of theory) might therefore involve such philosophical inquiry approaches *without* specifically drawing upon empirical (research) or experiential (expert) approaches. Indeed, some might argue that as a theory is an *expression* of how things are in reality, it cannot itself be observed and measured. Measuring programme outcomes that are the result of the application of a theory are not quite the same thing as evaluating the theory itself. Those (including those in nursing) who see theory evaluation as at least in part a rigorous philosophical endeavour might well reject as naive Weiss's (1998) view presented above, that such approaches are 'offhand' and 'informal' methods that lack rigor.

While the evaluative research orientation has existed for many decades, this tended to be a small sector in the wider world of evaluation. However, the increasing demands for evaluation based upon sound evidence changed all that. It is now increasingly recognised that a research orientation is a necessary underpinning for effective policy, programme and practice evaluation.

Many of the developments in evaluation research emphasise the predominant concerns of policy or programme evaluation. The impact of evaluation research (or evaluative research) on *theory* evaluation has thus far been limited. However, one interesting development in the increasing orientation towards research as an approach to evaluation is the focus upon theory and its place in programmes and practices that are being evaluated. Essentially the perspective is as follows: all policies and practice, and all intervention programmes, are to a greater or lesser extent theory driven. While some do not even acknowledge theory and it has to be sought out as an implicit underlying guiding influence, other programmes very overtly state the theory that is intended to drive them in each instance. It therefore becomes essential to focus upon theory, to identify the guiding theory and evaluate its impact upon the policy, practice or programme. Therefore, evaluative research increasingly takes on board the importance of theories that guide programmes, and incorporate theory evaluation within its remit.

Summative and formative evaluation

We have assumed that the issue of research evaluation versus non-research evaluation is a simple one of opposing poles. However, matters are a bit more complex than this. As indicated above, evaluation that we might term non-research evaluation can extend from little more than common sense value judgements to approaches that involve rigorous methods of philosophical inquiry.

Similarly, research evaluation can extend across its own continuum. This is to some extent a function of whether the disquiet is only with the more traditional concerns of policy or programme or practice intervention *outcomes*, or extends to concerns with the *processes* involved. It is also a function of whether the orientation is *formative* (to do with ongoing processes and changing things in response to emerging issues) or *summative* (to do with final positions on evaluation). It may seem that formative and process issues are the same thing as they are concerned with programme activities and practices. Similarly, it may seem that summative and outcome issues are the same thing as they are concerned with end points. However, the formative orientation involves an active interaction between evaluation and programme improvement that is more than passively evaluating the processes on an ongoing basis. On its side, the summative orientation presents not just outcome information but a final account of the processes, their formative refinement and shaping *and* the final outcome as measured against those that had been aimed for. Furthermore, because the research orientations addressing these different concerns (process and formative on one side, summative and outcomes on the other) may by necessity be different, there is a continuum here also. Figure 9.3 outlines the range of concerns and the different orientations that might emerge.

One further subtlety may be noted from Figure 9.3, particularly in respect of the research orientation that is more directed towards the formative and process issues. There is a sense in which the more traditional orientation toward summative and outcomes matters assumes that anticipated outcomes (those being aimed for) are given. In fact, these are often linked to the values of some powerful or influential group. The more interactive research orientation that attends to formative and process concerns tends to recognise that there may be other groups, other stakeholders, with different values. Their interests, and their aspirations in respect of outcomes, should also be taken into account. Increasingly there is a recognition that those phenomena that are being evaluated (whether they are an overall national health policy, or a specific theory that informs nursing practice) must take account of all stakeholders in the situation.

There may of course be different stakeholders concerned with nursing theory. Some of these theories have been designed to inform nursing management and leadership, others to inform or guide education and/or research, and yet others are intended to be specifically practice theories (in the sense that they are intended to inform clinical nursing practice). It may be that the reader will extend her or his study into such wider considerations subsequently. However, as we have indicated earlier, this book is intended to present vital notes on theory for students and practitioners rather than being a more advanced aid to postgraduate study. In this book, and in this chapter, our main stakeholders are the nurses, and of course their patients. Also important are the other members of the healthcare team, who may not necessarily share the same theoretical perspectives as nurses. It is important that these stakeholders' interests are addressed in the theory. In the context intended here, the theory is *nursing* theory, and more specifically, a theory that is intended to inform and guide clinical nurse–patient practice. This capacity to reflect key stakeholders' interests is therefore an additional dimension in our unfolding set of such dimensions, represented as the eleventh point in Table 9.4.

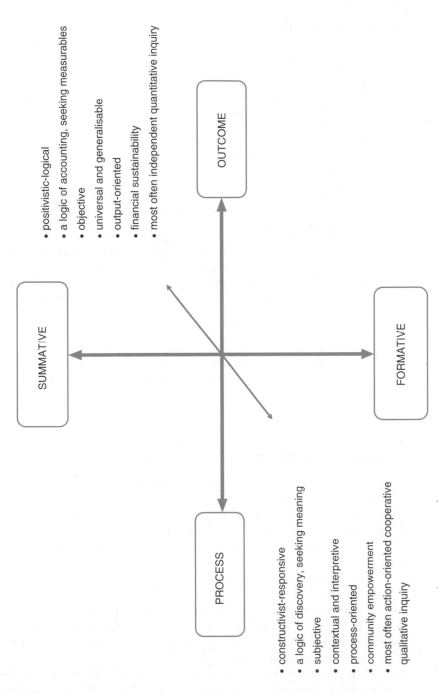

Figure 9.3 Evaluation as research: orientations.

- positivistic-logical
- a logic of accounting, seeking measurables
- objective
- universal and generalisable
- output-oriented
- financial sustainability
- most often independent quantitative inquiry

OUTCOME

SUMMATIVE

FORMATIVE

PROCESS

- constructivist-responsive
- a logic of discovery, seeking meaning
- subjective
- contextual and interpretive
- process-oriented
- community empowerment
- most often action-oriented cooperative qualitative inquiry

Table 9.4 The evaluation dimensions IV.

A good or worthy theory will:
1 be expressed in precise, clear and operational terms that allow us to test it *(Parsimony and Testability)*
2 withstand challenges to refute or falsify it, while being open to or facilitating such challenges *(Defeasibility)*
3 present, on the basis of the latter, the best available knowledge on the particular topic at the particular time *(Evidence and Justified True Belief)*
4 organise and express this knowledge in such a way that it (the theory) describes, and/or explains, and/or predicts phenomena and the relationships or links between them *(Coherence and Consistency)*
5 be useful or have utility in the practice of nursing *(Relevance and Utility)*
6 where it (the theory) *does* have utility for nursing, furthermore have withstood the challenges to its predictive powers consistently to the point where there is confidence in utilising it to *prescribe* nursing actions *(Prescriptive Value)*
7 identify or underpin certain standards and descriptors that pertain to quality of nursing care *(Quality Enhancement)*
8 contain within it a sense or essential nature that conveys its value as a source of nursing insight, a sense in which it illuminates nursing or a part of the nursing world *(Meaningfulness)*
9 be established upon a dynamic orientation that assumes testing as an *ongoing* commitment *(Dynamism)*
10 reflects a creative unfoldment that provides new and original meaning as opposed to simply restating current knowledge *(Originality)*
11 address the needs of nursing staff for guidance and as a consequence address the needs of those they are caring for *(Stakeholder Interests)*

Activity 4: Stakeholders

Earlier we considered different evaluation orientations:

* evaluation by research
* evaluation by experience and expertise
* evaluation by rational processes and critical reasoning.

All of these might (and often do) take place without the involvement of stakeholders.

Briefly review the literature on stakeholder involvement in evaluation. The areas of participatory evaluation (Patton 2002), empowerment evaluation and action research (any recent source) may prove useful starting points.

Consider how stakeholders might be involved in each of the three evaluation orientations listed above. Try to list at least three examples of involvement for each evaluation type.

Evaluation frameworks

We might have approached this project in a different way. We might have paid more attention to what might be termed seminal or influential contributions to the theory evaluation literature. Then drawing from one of these, or perhaps attempting to synthesise a new framework for evaluation from all or some of them, we might have proceeded to identify a means by which we could evaluate theories.

Instead, we have taken a different route. We have proceeded to consider the terminologies involved, the nature of knowledge to be evaluated as part of theory, the essential differences between theory testing and theory evaluation, and the different evaluation orientations – including research, non-research and other rational approaches. It will be clear to you that as we have proceeded through the chapter we identified dimensions of what we might expect a 'good' theory to be like. These are in fact the issues or items that we would use in our evaluation of theories and their contribution to nursing.

That is not to say that we should ignore the important contributions of the seminal or key contributions (mostly North American in orientation). Indeed, we can draw upon these contributions. For example, one particular aspect that has not come up in our own progression is what might be termed the scope of a theory, that is, the extent to which it addresses the range of issues that may be important in a nursing theory. This may involve considering scope and range as involving slightly different dimensions.

As can be seen in Figure 9.4, there are senses in which the theory may extend along a dimension of scope, from abstract concerns about the profession as a whole (as in universal aspects of nursing reflected in grand theory) to more concrete concerns concerning specific issues (as in hypotheses that may be tested). In effect, this is the broad scope of nursing theory extending from grand theory or macro theory through middle range theory to more operational practice theory (hypotheses or micro theory) that we discussed in Chapter 2.

On a different dimension, we can see in Figure 9.4 the range of theory as extending from a narrow concern with a specific aspect of nursing to a broader concern that encompasses the full range of nursing concerns. At its most all-inclusive, this might be seen as including the full range of the elements within the nursing metaparadigm as proposed by Fawcett (2005). That is, a mapping of the central elements that mark the parameters or essential concerns of the discipline, including:

- persons or human beings (singly, in small groupings in communities, or in whole societies);

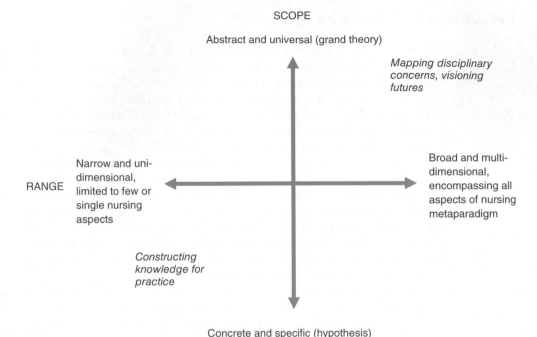

Figure 9.4 Range and scope of theory.

- environment (within which nursing takes place – encompassing physical, social and ecological environments);
- health (being the domain of concern within which nursing and other healthcare activities take place);
- nursing (which in this context is not the discipline, which is designated in the title nursing metaparadigm, but rather the activities that occur in nursing acts).

We can derive from this latter discussion an additional twelfth dimension that may assist with our evaluation of theory, presented as item 12 in Table 9.5, that is, the scope and range of a theory and the appropriateness of this in the particular instance.

At this point we have identified twelve dimensions or concerns that might be addressed in evaluating a theory. These are presented as a tentative listing that may not be appropriate in their entirety in all circumstances. Thus, if we are addressing theory that is – in terms of the twelfth of these dimensions (scope and range) – largely in the nature of a grand theory, it is unlikely that we will be concerned with the dimensions of testability and defeasibility. Such abstract theoretical statements would not be testable in that way.

Table 9.5 The evaluation dimensions V.

A good or worthy theory will:

1 be expressed in precise, clear and operational terms that allow us to test it *(Parsimony and Testability)*

2 withstand challenges to refute or falsify it, while being open to or facilitating such challenges *(Defeasibility)*

3 present, on the basis of the latter, the best available knowledge on the particular topic at the particular time *(Evidence and Justified True Belief)*

4 organise and express this knowledge in such a way that it (the theory) describes, and/or explains, and/or predicts phenomena and the relationships or links between them *(Coherence and Consistency)*

5 be useful or have utility in the practice of nursing *(Relevance and Utility)*

6 where it (the theory) *does* have utility for nursing, furthermore have withstood the challenges to its predictive powers consistently to the point where there is confidence in utilising it to *prescribe* nursing actions *(Prescriptive Value)*

7 identify or underpin certain standards and descriptors that pertain to quality of nursing care *(Quality Enhancement)*

8 contain within it a sense or essential nature that conveys its value as a source of nursing insight, a sense in which it illuminates nursing or a part of the nursing world *(Meaningfulness)*

9 be established upon a dynamic orientation that assumes testing as an *ongoing* commitment *(Dynamism)*

10 reflects a creative unfoldment that provides new and original meaning as opposed to simply restating current knowledge *(Originality)*

11 address the needs of nursing staff for guidance and as a consequence address the needs of those they are caring for *(Stakeholder Interests)*

12 depending upon its purpose, have an appropriate balance between the range of nursing concerns and the scope or level of abstraction it presents *(Scope and Range)*

The reader may note from the wide nursing literature on this topic of theory evaluation, two important considerations.

- First, there are so many learned statements on theory evaluation within the nursing literature (and we are almost unique in this respect) that there is a confusing array of frameworks to choose from. It seems that each endeavours to define the terms and parameters differently. Also it seems that each attempts to outdo the other in terms of increasing complexity. The student venturing into this maze may very quickly begin to develop a sense of inferiority in the face of such burgeoning sophistication.

- Second, despite the aforementioned confusing array of frameworks for theory evaluation, there is a sense in which there is also some common ground between them. This is illustrated in Table 9.6 which compares the twelve-item framework developed within this chapter with some of the more well-known alternatives. As will be

Table 9.6 Evaluation frameworks – differences and similarities.

	Fawcett (2005)	Walker and Avant (2005)	McKenna (1997)	McKenna and Slevin (2008)
1	Analysis: theory scope	Origins of theory	How the theory was developed	Parsimony and testability
2	Analysis: theory context	Meaning	How the theory is internally structured	Defeasibility
3	Analysis: theory content	Logical adequacy	How the theory may be used	Evidence and justified true belief
4	Evaluation: significance	Usefulness	How the theory influences knowledge development	Coherence and consistency
5	Evaluation: internal consistency	Generalisability	How the theory stands up to testing	Relevance and utility
6	Evaluation: parsimony	Parsimony		Prescriptive value
7	Evaluation: testability	Testability		Quality enhancement
8	Evaluation: empirical adequacy			Meaningfulness
9	Evaluation: pragmatic adequacy			Dynamism
10				Originality
11				Reflection of stakeholder interests
12				Scope and range

seen, while there are differences it is notable that there are also similarities across the four examples. For example, all include testability as an evaluation criterion. While only three of the four can be seen from the table to include parsimony, the fourth (McKenna's framework) includes it under the internal structure criterion.

Activity 5: Evaluating nursing theory

Take one of the examples from Table 9.6 – the Walker and Avant (2005) example. You may note incidentally, when you follow up their work, these authors claim to be doing theory analysis, suggesting that evaluation of theory is something that is different and can be found elsewhere. However, as other authors such as Meleis

(1985, 1991, 1997, 2007) and McEwen and Wills (2007) note, this is to a large extent a matter of semantics. What Walker and Avant are doing, others call evaluation.

Go to the section on theoretical analysis in the cited Walker and Avant text. Read this, paying particular attention to the seven elements of analysis (or evaluation) presented. Make brief definitions of the seven elements. When you have done this, review once again the twelve elements proposed in the current chapter (as outlined in Table 9.5 and Table 9.6). Reflect upon how you might use either of these frameworks.

Finally, identify some theory or theoretical framework you may have used in your practice. Try to identify a fairly straightforward example, avoiding some of the more esoteric cases found in the literature that might take you a month to understand, never mind evaluate. A good idea would be to think of something you may have used in your own practice – for example a theory that self-care promotes independence and wellbeing. Apply the twelve dimensions or elements from Table 9.5 to evaluate this example. Reflect on how many of the dimensions were relevant in evaluating your particular example, and the extent to which the theory measured up to the criteria in Table 9.5.

Conclusion

Let us make no mistake about it; this chapter, and indeed most of this book, is about the empirical form of knowledge. We have of course considered, briefly in Chapter 1 and in more detail in Chapter 3, the different patterns of knowing presented by Carper (1978). In this seminal work she proposed empirical, ethical, personal and aesthetic patterns of knowing. We have also recognised other frameworks that extend the sources of knowledge beyond the empirical. We have recognised – in this chapter and elsewhere – that as well as empirical methods we can also call upon logic and critical analysis to help construct, critique and even test knowledge.

However, the baseline fact remains. This book is about theory, and this chapter is about evaluation of theory. Theory – as we have construed it in this book – is a scientific construct. We have recognised, particularly in the opening chapter, that there are other ways in which the term theory may be used, and that it has specialist and more general everyday usages. We even recognised, back there, that some more traditional scientists reject the idea of theory being a part of science altogether! Still, the point remains: we are concerned with theory as a scientific construct. We are concerned with that knowledge form that is usually termed empirical (derived from observation and experience).

On this basis we have proceeded in this chapter towards exploring the issues concerned with evaluating theory in this context. We have furthermore proceeded as we progressed through the chapter to develop a twelve-point framework for evaluating theory. This also takes its position within the empirical orientation. The framework is only suited to evaluating theory in its sense as a scientific construct. It is best suited to evaluating the more operational middle range theory, and micro theory that is even more operational if not indeed at the level of testable hypotheses. It will also succeed in evaluating that theory we term grand theory in this book, although some of the more precise dimensions of the framework, such as theory testability, would not be relevant.

It is hoped that the framework will provide insight for our readers, or at least point them towards helpful resources elsewhere. However, in closing we would propose caution in assuming that theory evaluation is a sufficient test of nursing knowledge. Speaking of the wider patterns of knowing suggested by Carper (1978), Chinn and Kramer write:

> 'Empirics removed from the context of the whole of knowing produces control and manipulation. Ironically, these have been explicit traditional goals of the empiric sciences . . .
>
> 'Ethics removed from the context of the whole of knowing produces rigid doctrine and insensitivity to the rights of others. This happens when someone simply sets forth personal ideas concerning what is right or good . . .
>
> 'Personal knowing removed from the context of the whole of knowing produces isolation and self-distortion. When this happens, the self remains isolated, and knowledge of self comes only from what is known internally . . .
>
> 'Aesthetics removed from the context of the whole of knowing produces indulgence in self-serving expressions and lack of appreciation for the fullness of meaning in a context. Human actions emerge from and are represented by the tastes and desires of the individual alone, without taking into account the deep cultural meanings inherent in the art-act.'
>
> Chinn and Kramer (1999: 12–13)

Their text is for its greater part concerned with the empirical dimension and within this what they term critical reflection of theory (evaluation by another name). But they are of course right in recognising that, in nursing, knowing extends beyond the empirical. At the conclusion of this chapter, the reader might reflect upon the importance of not only evaluating theory but also thinking critically about the other patterns of knowing that inform our practice and how they too must be evaluated.

Summary

The chapter began with a recognition of the need for parsimony in theory, that being stated simply and in operational terms, theory can be adequately tested. The movement toward theory evaluation involved a consideration of terminology, including discussion of and clarification in respect of terms such as right, wrong, value, worth, standards and quality. The importance of establishing 'value' was introduced, and a critique of what we might mean by valuing theory was outlined. The characteristics of a theory were reviewed and expressed in terms of the attributes or dimensions of a 'good' theory. These attributes were explored as the basis for evaluating a theory. From this exploration a framework of twelve dimensions or criteria for testing a theory was developed and presented. The particular place of testing a theory was considered, and the relationship between theory evaluation and theory testing clarified. In conclusion, the importance of recognising theory as a scientific construct and theory evaluation as being limited to addressing such constructs was highlighted. It was recognised that there are other patterns of knowing in nursing – particularly those proposed by Carper (1978) and critiqued by Chinn and Kramer (1999). The chapter concluded by highlighting the importance of evaluating these other aspects of nursing knowledge.

References

Abdellah F.G., Beland I.L., Martin A. & Matheney R.V. (1960) *Patient Centred Approaches to Nursing*. New York: Macmillan.

Adam E.T. (1975) A conceptual model for nursing. *Canadian Nurse*, **71**, 40–43.

Adam E.T. (1980) *To be a Nurse*. New York: W.B. Saunders.

Aggleton P. & Chalmers C. (2000) *Nursing Models and Nursing Practice*, 2nd edition. Basingstoke, UK: Palgrave.

Ajzen I. (1998) *Attitudes, Personality and Behavior*. Chicago, IL: The Dorsey Press.

Alligood M.R. & Marriner Tomey A. (2002) *Nursing Theory: Utilization and Application*, 2nd edition. St Louis, MO: Mosby, Inc.

Alligood M.R. & Marriner Tomey A. (2006) *Nursing Theory: Utilization and Application*, 3rd edition. St Louis, MO: Mosby, Inc.

Anderson J.A. (2001) Understanding homeless adults by testing the theory of self care. *Nursing Science Quarterly*, **14**(1), 59–67.

Argyris C. & Schön D. (1974) *Theory in Practice*. London: Jossey-Bass.

Barnes P. (2004) The nurse clinician: a time to reflect qualification. Paper presented at NMC Post Registration Nursing Framework Consultation Conference, February.

Barnhart C.L. & Barnhart R.K. (1976) *The Worldbook Dictionary Field*. Chicago, IL: Enterprises Educational Corporation.

Barnum B. (1990) *Nursing Theory: Analysis, Application, Evaluation*, 3rd edition. Glenview, IL: Little, Brown.

Beauchamp T.L. & Childress J.F. (2001) *Principles of Biomedical Ethics*, 5th edition. Oxford, UK: Oxford University Press.

Beck U. (1992) *Risk Society: Towards a New Modernity*. London: Sage.

Beck U. (1999) *World Risk Society*. Malden, MA: Polity Press.

Beckstrand J. (1980) A critique of several conceptions of practice theory in nursing. *Research in Nursing and Health*, **3**(2), 69–80.

Benner P. (1983) Uncovering the knowledge embedded in clinical practice. *Image: the Journal of Nurse Scholarship*, **15**, 36–44.

Benner P. (1984) *From Novice to Expert: Excellence and Power in Clinical Nursing Practice*. Menlo Park, CA: Addison-Wesley.

Benner P. & Wrubel J. (1989) *The Primacy of Caring: Stress and Coping in Health and Illness*. Menlo Park, CA: Addison-Wesley.

Benner P., Hopper-Kyriakidis P. & Stannard D. (1999) *Clinical Wisdom and Interventions in Critical Care*. Philadelphia, PA: W.B. Saunders Company.

Bevis E.M. (1988) New directions for a new age. In National League for Nurses (ed.) *Curriculum Revolution*. New York: National League for Nurses.

Biddle B.J. & Thomas E.J. (1966) *Role Theory: Concepts and Research*. New York: John Wiley & Sons Inc.

Bishop S.M. (1986) History and philosophy of science. In Marriner A. (ed.) *Nursing Theorists and their Work*. St Louis, MO: Mosby, Inc.

Blumer H. (1969) *Symbolic Interactionism: Perspective and Method*. Englewood Cliffs, NJ: Prentice Hall.

BMA (British Medical Association) Health Policy & Economic Research Unit (2002) The future healthcare workforce – discussion paper 9. London: British Medical Association.

Bogdanovic A. (1989) Non-verbal communication. *Nursing Times*, **85**(1), 27–28.

Bohm D. (1980) *Wholeness and the Implicate Order*. London: Ark.

Bohm D. (1987) *Unfolding Meaning*. London: Routledge.

Bohm D. (1998a) On the relationships of science and art. In Bohm D. *On Creativity*. London: Routledge.

Bohm D (1998b) *On Creativity*. London: Routledge.

Boore J.R.P. (1978) *A Prescription for Recovery*. London: Royal College of Nursing.

Bourdieu P. (1977) *Outline of a Theory of Practice* (trans. R. Nice). Cambridge, UK: Cambridge University Press.

Bower P., Jerrim S. & Gask L. (2004) Primary care mental health workers: role expectations, conflict and ambiguity. *Health and Social Care in the Community*, **12**(4), 336–345.

Bridges J., Meyer J., Glynn M., Bentley J. & Reeves S. (2003) Interprofessional care co-ordinators: the benefits and tensions associated with a new role in UK acute health care. *International Journal of Nursing Studies*, **40**, 599–607.

Bronowski J. (2005) *The Ascent of Man*: the complete series digitally restored. London: BBC.

Buchan J. & Daz Pol M. (2002) Skill mix in the health care workforce: reviewing the evidence. *Bulletin of the World Health Organization*, **80**(7), 575–580.

Buchan J. & Seccombe I. (2003) *More Nurses Working Differently? A Review of the UK Nursing Labour Market 2002 to 2003*. London: Royal College of Nursing.

Burkeman O. (2005) Not even wrong. *The Guardian*, 19 September 2005.

Cabinet Office (1999) *Modernising Government*. London: The Stationery Office.

Cabinet Office (2001) *Better Policy Delivery and Design: a Discussion Paper*. London: The Stationery Office.

Cameron A. & Masterson A. (2000) Managing the unmanageable? Nurse executive directors and the new role in nursing. *Journal of Advanced Nursing*, **31**(5), 1081–1088.

Carper B.A. (1978) Fundamental patterns of knowing in nursing. *Advances in Nursing Science*, **1**(1), 13–23.

Carper B.A. (1992) Philosophical inquiry in nursing: an application. In Kikuchi J.F. & Simmons H. (eds) *Philosophic Inquiry in Nursing*. Newbury Park, CA: Sage.

Castledine G. (1986) A stress adaptation model. In Kershaw B. & Salvage J. (eds) *Models for Nursing*. Chichester, UK: John Wiley & Sons.

Castledine G. (2003) *Generalist and Specialist Nurses – Complementary or Conflicting Roles?* Edinburgh, UK: Scottish Executive.

Chalmers H. (1989) Theories and models of nursing and the nursing process. In Akinsanya J.A. (ed.) *Theories and Models of Nursing*. Edinburgh, UK: Churchill Livingstone.

Chambers M. (1995) Learning psychiatric nursing skills: the contribution of the ward environment. University of Ulster, Unpublished D.Phil thesis.

Chapman C.M. (1985) *Theory of Nursing: Practical Application*. London: Harper & Row.

Chapman P. (1990) A critical perspective. In Salvage J. & Kershaw B. (eds) *Models for Nursing 2*. London: Scutari Press.

Charlton A. (1980) *The Belcarra Park Site*. Publication no. 9. Burnaby, BC: Simon Fraser University.

Childers T. (1989) Evaluative research in the library and information field. *Library Trends*, **38**(2), 250–267.

Chinn P.L. & Kramer M.K. (1995) *Theory and Nursing: A Systematic Approach*, 4th edition. St Louis, MO: Mosby, Inc.

Chinn P.L. & Kramer M.K. (1999) *Theory and Nursing: Integrated Knowledge Development*, 5th edition. St Louis, MO: Mosby, Inc.

Chinn P.L. & Kramer M.K. (2004) *Integrated Knowledge Development in Nursing*, 6th edition. St Louis, MO: Mosby, Inc.

Clark J. (1986) A model for health visiting. In Kershaw B. & Salvage J. (eds) *Models for Nursing*. Chichester, UK: John Wiley & Sons.

Clarke M. (1986) Action and reflection: practice and theory in nursing. *Journal of Advanced Nursing*, **11**, 3–11.

Cohen D. & Prusak L. (2001) *In Good Company: How Social Capital Makes Organizations Work*. Boston, MA: Harvard Business School Press.

Collins W. (1992) *Death of an Angel*. London: Pan Macmillan.

Conway M.E. (1978) Theoretical approaches to the study of roles. In Hardy M.E. & Conway M.E. (eds) *Role Theory: Perspectives for Health Professionals*. New York: Appleton-Century-Crofts.

Craig S.L. (1980) Theory development and its relevance for nursing. *Journal of Advanced Nursing*, **5**, 349–355.

Cutcliffe J.R. & McKenna H.P. (2005) *The Essential Concepts of Nursing: Building Blocks for Practice*. London: Elsevier.

Daly W.M. & Carnwell R. (2003) Nursing roles and levels of practice: a framework for differentiating between elementary, specialist and advancing nursing practice. *Journal of Clinical Nursing*, **12**, 158–167.

Davies C. (1995) *Gender and the Professional Predicament in Nursing*. Buckingham, UK: Open University Press.

Davies C. (2001) Changing practice in health care (editorial). *Postgraduate Medical Journal*, **77**(905), 145–147.

Davies H., Nutley S. & Smith P. (2000) *What works? Evidence-based Policy and Practice in Public Services*. Bristol, UK: Policy Press.

Denner S. (1995) Extending professional practice: benefits and pitfalls. *Nursing Times*, **91**(14), 27.

Dickoff J. & James P. (1968) A theory of theories: a position paper. *Nursing Research*, **17**(3), 197–203.

Dickoff J. & James P. (1971) Clarity to what end? *Nursing Research*, **20**(6), 499–502.

Dickoff J. & James P. (1992) Correspondence. In Nicholl L. (ed.) *Perspectives on Nursing Theory*, 2nd edition. New York: J.B. Lippincott.

Diers D. (1979) *Research in Nursing Practice*. Philadelphia, PA: J.B. Lippincott.

DoH (Department of Health) (1994) *Working in Partnership. The report from the Mental Health Review Team*. London: HMSO.

Duldt B. & Griffin K. (1985) *Theoretical Perspectives for Nursing*. Boston, MA: Little, Brown.

Edwards S. & Liaschenko J. (2003) On the quest for a theory of nursing. *Nursing Philosophy*, **4**, 1–3.

Ellis R. (1969) The practitioner as theorist. *American Journal of Nursing*, **69**, 1434–1438.

Ellis R. (1970) Values and vicissitudes of the scientist nurse. *Nursing Research*, **19**(5), 440–445.

Emden C. (1991) Ways of knowing in nursing. In Gray G. & Pratt R. (eds) *Towards a Discipline of Nursing*, pp. 11–30. Edinburgh, UK: Churchill Livingstone.

Engel G.L. (1977) The need for a new medical model: a challenge for biomedicine. *Science*, **196**(4286), 129–136.

Entwhistle V.A., Sheldon T.A., Sowden A. & Watt I.S. (1998) Evidence-informed patient choice: practical issues of involving patients in decisions about health care technologies. *International Journal of Technology Assessment in Health Care*, **14**, 212–225.

Erickson H., Tomlin E. & Swain M. (1983) *Modelling and Role Modelling*. Lexington, SC: Pine Press.

Ersser S. (2006) What's in the black box? Past and future perspectives on nursing as a therapeutic activity. Interpersonal Relationships in Nursing Conference, Aarhus, Denmark: August 2006.

Ewens A. (2003) Changes in nursing identities: supporting a successful tradition. *Journal of Nursing Management*, **11**, 224–228.

Fawcett J. (1989, 1995) *Analysis and Evaluation of Conceptual Models of Nursing*, 2nd & 3rd editions. Philadelphia, PA: F.A. Davis.

Fawcett J. (1999) The *The Relationship of Theory and Research*, 3rd edition. Philadelphia, PA: F. A. Davis.

Fawcett J. (2005) *Contemporary Nursing Knowledge: Analysis and Evaluation of Nursing Models and Theories*, 2nd edition. Philadelphia, PA: F.A. Davis.

Fawcett J. (2006) Conceptual Models, Theories, and Research. Lecture delivered at University of Ulster, Jordanstown, Northern Ireland, March 2006.

Fawcett J. & Downs F.S. (1992) *The Relationship of Theory and Research*, 2nd edition. Philadelphia, PA: F.A. Davis.

Feyerabend P. (1977) Consolidation for the specialist. In Lakatos I. & Musgrave A. (eds) *Criticism and the Growth of Knowledge*. Cambridge, UK: Cambridge University Press.

Fitzpatrick J.J. (1982) In Fitzpatrick J.J., Whall A.L., Johnston R.L. & Floyd J.A. (eds) *Nursing Models: Applications to Psychiatric Mental Health Nursing*. Bowie, MD: Brady & Co.

Fitzpatrick J.J. & Whall A.L. (1983) *Conceptual Models of Nursing: Analysis and Application*. Bowie, MD: Brady & Co.

Fosbinder D. (1994) Patient perceptions of nursing care: an emerging theory of interpersonal competence. *Journal of Advanced Nursing*, **20**, 1085–1093.

Freud S. (1949) *An Outline of Psychoanalysis*. New York: W.W. Norton.

Friend B. (1990) Working at health. *Nursing Times*, **86**(16), 21.

Gadamer H.-G. (1989) *Truth and Method*. London: Sheed & Ward.

Gadow S. (1990) Response to 'personal knowing: evolving research and practice'. *Scholarly Inquiry in Nursing Practice*, **4**(2), 167–170.

George J. (ed.) (1985) *Nursing Theories: The Base for Professional Practice*. Englewood Cliffs, NJ: Prentice Hall.

George J. (ed.) (1995) *Nursing Theories: The Base for Professional Practice*, 3rd edition. Englewood Cliffs, NJ: Prentice Hall.

George J. (ed.) (2001) *Nursing Theories: The Base for Professional Practice*, 5th edition. Englewood Cliffs, NJ: Prentice Hall.

Giddens A. (1999) *Runaway World: How Globalisation is Reshaping our Lives*. London: Profile Books.

Girot E. (1990) Discussing nursing theory. *Senior Nurse*, **10**(6), 16–19.

Glaser B.J. & Strauss A.L. (1967) *Discovery of Grounded Theory: Strategies for Qualitative Research*. Chicago, IL: Aldine Publishing.

Gortner S.R. (1993) Nursing's syntax revisited: a critique of philosophies said to influence nursing theories. *International Journal of Nursing Studies*, **30**(6), 477–488.

Grahame P.J. (1987) Backchat. *Nursing Times*, **83**(16), 22.

Greaves F. (1984) *Nurse Education and The Curriculum: A Curricular Model*, pp. 88–93. London: Croom Helm.

Green C. (1988) The development of a conceptual model for mental handicap nursing practice in the UK. *Nurse Education Today*, **8**, 9–17.

Habermas J. (1971) *Knowledge and Human Interests*. Boston, MA: Beacon Press.

Hall L. (1959) *Nursing – What is it?* Virginia: Virginia State Nurses Association. Winter.

Halsey S. (1978) The queen bee syndrome: one solution to role conflict for nurse managers. In Hardy M.E. & Conway M.E. (eds) *Role Theory: Perspectives for Health Professionals*. New York: Appleton-Century-Crofts.

Hamans G.C. (1966) Norms and behaviour. In Biddle B.J. & Thomas E.J. (eds) *Role Theory: Concepts and Research*. New York: John Wiley & Sons Inc.

Hardy L.K. (1986) Janforum. Identifying the place of theoretical frameworks in an evolving discipline. *Journal of Advanced Nursing*, **11**, 103–107.

Hardy M.E. (1978) Perspectives on knowledge and role theory. In Hardy M.E. & Conway M.E. (eds) *Role Theory: Perspectives for Health Professionals*. New York: Appleton-Century-Crofts.

Hawkett S. (1989) A model marriage. *Nursing Times*, **85**(1), 61–62.

Henderson V. (1966) *The Nature of Nursing: A Definition and its Implications for Practice, Education and Research*. London: Collier Macmillan.

Henderson V. & Harmer B. (1955) *Textbook of the Principles and Practices of Nursing*, 5th edition. New York: Macmillan.

Hinshaw A.S. (1978) Role attitudes: a measurement problem. In Hardy M.E. & Conway M.E. (eds) *Role Theory: Perspectives for Health Professionals*. New York: Appleton-Century-Crofts.

Hoff L.A. (1995) *People in Crisis: Understanding and Helping*, 4th edition. San Francisco, CA: Jossey-Bass.

Holden R.J. (1990) Models, muddles and medicine. *International Journal of Nursing Studies*, **27**(3), 223–234.

Houlihan P.J. (1986) The marketing of nursing jargon. *Canadian Nurse*, February, 21–22.

House E.R. & Howe K.R. (1999) *Values in Evaluation and Social Research*. Thousand Oaks, CA: Sage.

Huch M.H. (1995) Nursing and the next millennium. *Nursing Science Quarterly*, **8**(1), 38–44.

Husserl E. (1962) *Ideas: General Introduction to Pure Phenomenology*. New York: Collier.

Ingersoll G. (2000) Evidence-based nursing: what it is and isn't. *Nursing Outlook*, **48**, 151–152.

Jack B., Hendry C. & Topping A. (2004) Third year student nurses' perceptions of the role and impact of Clinical Nurse Specialists: a multi-centred descriptive study. *Clinical Effectiveness in Nursing*, **8**, 39–46.

Jackson M. (1986) On maps and models. *Senior Nurse*, **5**(4), 24–26.

Jacox A.K. (1974) Theory construction in nursing: an overview. *Nursing Research*, **23**(1), 4–13.

Jacox A.K. & Webster G. (1992) Competing theories of science. In Nicoll L. (ed.) *Perspectives on Nursing Theory*, 2nd edition. New York: J.B. Lippincott.

Jensen A.R. (1973) Race, intelligence and genetics: the differences are real. *Psychology Today*, **12**, 80–86.

Johnson D.E. (1959) The nature of a science of nursing. *Nursing Outlook*, **7**, 291–294.

Johnson D.E. (1968) Theory in nursing: borrowed and unique. *Nursing Research*, **17**(3), 206–209.

Johnson M. (1983) Some aspects of the relation between theory and research in nursing. *Journal of Advanced Nursing*, **8**, 21–28.

Kahn R.L., Wolfe D.M., Quinn R.P., Diedrick Snoek J. & Rosenthal R.A. (1966) Adjustment to role conflict and ambiguity in organizations. In Biddle B.J. & Thomas E.J. (eds) *Role Theory: Concepts and Research*. New York: John Wiley & Sons Inc.

Kendall L. & Lissauer T. (2003) *The Future Health Worker*. London: IPPR.

Kerlinger F.N.B. (1986) *Foundations of Behavioural Research*, 3rd edition. New York: Holt, Rinehart & Winston.

Kim H.S. (1983) *The Nature of Theoretical Thinking in Nursing*. Norwalk, CT: Appleton-Century-Crofts.

Kim H.S. (1989) Theoretical thinking in nursing. In Akinsanya J. (ed.) *Recent Advances in Nursing*, **24**, 106–122.

King I. (1968) A conceptual frame of reference for nursing. *Nursing Research*, **17**(1), 27–31.

King I. (1971) *Toward a Theory for Nursing: General Concepts of Human Behaviour*. New York: John Wiley & Sons Inc.

King I. (1981) *A Theory of Nursing: Systems, Concepts, Process*. New York: John Wiley & Sons Inc.

Kitson A.L. (1984) Unpublished paper. University of Ulster, Coleraine, Northern Ireland.

Kolcaba K. (2001) Evolution of the mid range theory of comfort for outcomes research. *Nursing Outlook*, **49**(2), 86–92.

Kuhn T. (1962, 1970) *The Structure of Scientific Revolutions*, 1st & 2nd editions. Chicago: Chicago University Press.

Kuhn T.S. (1977) *The Structure of Scientific Revolutions*, 3rd edition. Chicago: Chicago University Press.

Lambert V.A. & Lambert C.E. (2001) Literature review of role stress/strain on nurses: an international perspective. *Nursing Health Science*, **3**(3), 161–172.

Lane P., McKenna H.P., Ryan A.A. & Fleming P. (2003) The experience of the family caregiver's role: a qualitative study. *Research and Theory for Nursing Practice*, **17**(2), 137–152.

Last T. & Self N. (1994) The expanded role of the nurse in intensive care. In Hunt G. & Wainwright P. (eds) *Expanding the Role of the Nurse: The Scope of Professional Practice*. Oxford, UK: Blackwell Scientific Publications.

Laudan L. (1977) *Progress and its Problems: Towards a Theory of Scientific Growth*. Berkeley, CA: University of California Press.

le Carré, John (2001) *The Constant Gardener*. London: Hodder & Stoughton.

Leininger M.M. (1978) *Transcultural Nursing: Concepts, Theories, and Practices*. New York: John Wiley & Sons Inc.

Levenson B. & Vaughan B. (1999) *Developing New Roles in Practice: An Evidence Based Guide*. Sheffield, UK: University of Sheffield.

Levine M.E. (1966) Adaptation and assessment: a rationale for nursing intervention. *American Journal of Nursing*, **66**(11), 2450–2453.

Levine M.E. (1994) Some further thoughts on the ethics of nursing rhetoric. In Kikuchi J.F. & Simmons H. (eds) *Developing a Philosophy of Nursing*. Thousand Oaks, CA: Sage.

Lyotard J.-F. (1984) *The Postmodern Condition: A Report on Knowledge*. Minneapolis, MN: Minnesota University Press.

Maloney E. (1984) Theoretical approaches. In Beck C.A., Rawlings R.P. & Williams S.R. (eds) *Mental Health Psychiatric Nursing: A Holistic Life Cycle Approach*. St Louis, MO: Mosby, Inc.

Mansfield E. (1980) A conceptual framework for psychiatric mental health care nursing. *Journal of Psychiatric Nursing and Mental Health Services*, **18**(4), 34–41.

Maslow A.H. (1954) *Motivation and Personality*. New York: Harper & Row.

McCaughan E.M. & McKenna H.P (2007) Information-seeking behaviour of men newly diagnosed with cancer. *Journal of Clinical Nursing*, **15**(2), 1–9.

McEwen M. & Wills, E.M. (2007) *Theoretical Basis for Nursing*, 2nd edition. Philadelphia, PA: Lippincott, Williams &Wilkins.

McFarlane J.K. (1982) Nursing: A Paradigm of Caring. Unpublished paper. Ethical Issues in Caring. University of Manchester, UK.

McFarlane J.K. (1986) The value of models of care. In Kershaw B. & Salvage J. (eds) *Models for Nursing*. Chichester, UK: John Wiley & Sons.

McGee P. & Castledine G. (1999) A survey of specialist and advanced nursing practice in the UK. *British Journal of Nursing*, **8**(16), 1074–1078.

McKenna H.P. (1990) A pill for every ill. *Nursing Times*, **86**(10): 28–31.

McKenna H.P. (1994) *Nursing Theories and Quality of Care*. Aldershot, UK: Avebury Press.

McKenna H.P. (1995) Nursing skill mix substitutions and quality of care: an exploration of assumptions from the research literature. *Journal of Advanced Nursing*, **21**, 452–459.

McKenna H.P. (1997) *Nursing Theories and Models*. London: Routledge.

McKenna H.P. (2004) 'Role drift' to unlicensed assistants: risks to quality and safety. Editorial. *Quality and Safety in Health Care*, **13**(6), 410–411.

McKenna H.P., Keeney S. & Bradley M. (2003) Generic and specialist nursing roles in the community: an investigation of professional and lay views. *Health and Social Care in the Community*, **11**(6), 537–545.

McKenna H.P., McCann S.M., McCaughan E.M. & Keeney S.R. (2004) The role of an outreach oncology nurse practitioner: a case study evaluation. *European Journal of Oncology Nursing*, **8**(1), 66–77.

McKenna H.P., Keeney S.R., Hasson F., Richey R., Sinclair M. & Poulton B. (2005) *Innovative Roles in Nursing and Midwifery*. Belfast: Northern Ireland Practice and Education Council for Nursing and Midwifery.

McSherry R., Simmons M. & Pearce P. (2002) An introduction to evidence-informed nursing. In McSherry R., Simmons M. & Abbott P. (eds) *Evidence-Informed Nursing: A Guide for Nurses*. London: Routledge.

Meave M.K. (1994) The carrier bag theory of nursing practice. *Advances in Nursing Science*, **16**(4), 9–22.

Meleis A.I. (1985, 1991) *Theoretical Nursing: Development and Progress,* 1st & 2nd editions. Philadelphia, PA: J.B. Lippincott.

Meleis A.I. (1997) *Theoretical Nursing: Development and Progress,* 3rd edition. New York: J.B. Lippincott.

Meleis A.I. (2007) *Theoretical Nursing: Development and Progress,* 4th edition. Philadelphia, PA: Lippincott Williams & Wilkins.

Menzies I.E.P. (1960) A case study in the functioning of social systems as a defence against anxiety: a report of a study of the nursing service of a general hospital. *Human Relations*, **13**(2), 95–121.

Mercer R.T. (1995) *Becoming a Mother: Research from Rubin to the Present*. New York: Springer.

Merton R.K. (1966) Instability and articulation in the role-set. In Biddle B.J. & Thomas E.J. (eds) *Role Theory: Concepts and Research*. New York: John Wiley & Sons Inc.

Merton R.K. (1968) *Social Theory and Social Structure*. New York: Free Press.

Merton T. (1969) *My Argument with the Gestapo: A Macaronic Journal*. New York: Doubleday & The Abbey of Gethsemane.

Midgely C. (1988) The use of models for nursing within midwifery training hospitals in England. Huddersfield Polytechnic, Huddersfield, UK. Unpublished paper.

Miller A. (1985) The relationship between nursing theory and nursing practice. *Journal of Advanced Nursing*, **10**, 414–424.

Miller A. (1989) Theory to practice: implementation in the clinical setting. In Jolley M. & Allen P. (eds) *Current Issues in Nursing*, pp. 47–65. London: Chapman & Hall.

Minshull J., Ross K. & Turner J. (1986) The human needs model of nursing. *Journal of Advanced Nursing*, **11**, 643–649.

Mishel M.H. (1990) Reconceptualisation of the uncertainty in illness theory. *Image: the Journal of Nurse Scholarship*, **22**, 256–261.

Mitchell R.G. (1986) *Essential Psychiatric Nursing*. Edinburgh, UK: Churchill Livingstone.

Moody L.E. (1990) *Advancing Nursing Science through Research,* volume 1. Newbury Park, CA: Sage.

Morse J.M. (1995) Exploring the theoretical basis of nursing using advanced techniques of concept analysis. *Advances in Nursing Science*, **17**(3), 31–46.

Muir Gray J.A. (1997) *Evidence-Based Health Care*. Edinburgh, UK: Churchill Livingstone.

Neuman B. (1995) *The Neuman Systems Model*, 3rd edition. Norwalk, CT: Appleton & Lange.

Neuman B. & Young R.J. (1972) A model for teaching total person approach to patient problems. *Nursing Research*, **21**(3), 264.

Newman M.A. (1979) *Theory Development in Nursing*, 3rd edition. Philadelphia, PA: F.A. Davis.

Nicholl L.H. (1992) *Perspectives on Nursing Theory*, 2nd edition. Boston, MA: Little Brown & Co (reprinted from *Image*, **9**(3), 59–63).

Nightingale F. (1859/1980) *Notes on Nursing: What It Is and What It Is Not*. Edinburgh, UK: Churchill Livingstone.

Nolan M. & Grant G. (1992) Mid-range theory building and the nursing theory-practice gap: a respite care case study. *Journal of Advanced Nursing*, **17**, 217–223.

OECD (Organisation for Economic Cooperation and Development) (2001) *Social Sciences for Knowledge and Decision Making*. Paris: OECD.

Orem D.E. (1958) *Nursing: Concepts of Practice*. New York: McGraw Hill.

Orem D.E. (1959) *Guides for Development of Curriculae for the Education of Practical Nurses*. Washington, DC: US Dept of Health, Education and Welfare.

Orem D.E. (1980) *Nursing: Concepts of Practice*, 2nd edition. New York: McGraw Hill.

Orem D.E. (1985) *Nursing: Concepts of Practice*, 3rd edition. New York: McGraw Hill.

Orem D.E. (1995) *Nursing: Concepts of Practice*, 5th edition. New York: McGraw Hill.

Orlando I. (1961) *The Dynamic Nurse Patient Relationship: Function, Process, and Principles*. New York: G.P. Putnam & Sons.

Parse R.R. (1981) *Man-Living-Health: A Theory of Nursing*. New York: John Wiley & Sons Inc.

Parse R.R. (1987) *Nursing Science: Major Paradigms, Theories and Critiques*. Philadelphia, PA: W.B. Saunders.

Parsons T. (1952) *The Social System*. London: Tavistock Publications.

Patterson J.G. & Zderad L.T. (1976) *Humanistic Nursing*. New York: John Wiley & Sons Inc.

Patton M.Q. (2002) *Qualitative Research and Evaluation Methods*. Thousand Oaks, CA: Sage.

Pawson R. (2001) *Evidence Based Policy: II The Promise of Realist Synthesis*. London: ESRC UK Centre for Evidence Based Policy and Practice, University of London.

Pawson R. (2002) Evidence-based policy: in search of a method. *Evaluation*, **8**(2), 157–181.

Pearson A. (2003) Multidisciplinary nursing: re-thinking role boundaries. *Journal of Clinical Nursing*, **12**, 625–629.

Peierls P. (1960) Wolfgang Ernst Pauli, 1900–1958. *Biographical Memoirs of Fellows of the Royal Society*, **5**(February 1960), 174–192.

Peplau H.E. (1952) *Interpersonal Relations in Nursing*. New York: G.P. Putnam & Sons.

Peplau H.E. (1962) Interpersonal techniques: the crux of nursing. *American Journal of Nursing*, **62**, 50–54.

Peplau H.E. (1965) The heart of nursing: interpersonal relations. *Canadian Nurse*, **61**, 273–275.

Peplau H.E. (1987) Nursing science: a historical perspective. In Parse R.R. (ed.) *Nursing Science: Major Paradigms, Theories and Critiques*. Philadelphia, PA: W.B. Saunders Company.

Peplau H.E. (1988) The art and science of nursing: similarities, differences and relations. *Nursing Science Quarterly*, **1**, 8–15.

Peplau H.E. (1992) Interpersonal relations: a theoretical framework for application in nursing practice. *Nursing Science Quarterly*, **5**, 13–18.

Peplau H.E. (1995a) Schizophrenia. Conference Presentation, Annual Conference, University of Ulster, Northern Ireland.

Peplau H.E. (1995b) Foreword. In Farren G.C.J., Herth K.A. & Popovich J.M. (eds) *Hope and Hopelessness: Critical Clinical Constructs*. Thousand Oaks, CA: Sage.

Peterson S.J. & Bredow T.S. (2004) *Middle Range Theories: Application to Nursing Theory*. Philadelphia, PA: Lippincott Williams & Wilkins.

Pierce C.S. (1957) *Essays in the Philosophy of Science*. Indianapolis, IN: Bobbs-Merrill.

Pirsig R.M. (1974) *Zen and the Art of Motorcycle Maintenance*. London: Bodley Head.

Pirsig R.M. (1993) *Lila, An Inquiry into Morals*. London: Black Swan.

Polanyi M. (1958) *Personal Knowledge: Towards A Post-Critical Philosophy*. Chicago: Chicago University Press.

Polanyi M. (1966) *The Tacit Dimension*, 1st edition. London: Doubleday.

Polanyi M. (1967) *The Tacit Dimension*, 2nd edition. London: Routledge & Kegan Paul.

Popper K. (1963, 1965) *Conjectures and Refutations: The Growth of Scientific Knowledge*, 1st & 2nd editions. New York: Harper & Row.

Popper K. (1989) *Conjectures and Refutations: The Growth of Scientific Knowledge*, 5th edition. London: Routledge.

Popper K. (1994) *The Myth of the Framework: In Defence of Science and Rationality*. (Edited by M.A. Notturno). New York: Routledge.

Popper K. (1999) *All Life is Problem Solving*. London: Routledge.

Rambo B.J. (1984) *Adaptation Nursing: Assessment and Intervention*. Philadelphia, PA: W.B. Saunders Company.

Read S., Lloyd Jones M., Collins K., McDonnell A., Jones R., Doyle L. et al. (2001) *Exploring new roles in practice: implications of developments within the clinical team (ENRiP)*. School of Health and Related Research (ScHARR), University of Sheffield, Sheffield www.shef.ac.uk/content/1/c6/33/98/enrip.pdf – accessed June 2004.

Reed P.G. (1989) Nursing theorizing as an ethical endeavour. *Advances in Nursing Science*, **11**(3), 1–9.

Reynolds P.D. (1971) *A Primer for Theory Construction.* Indianapolis, IN: Bobbs-Merrill.

Rhyl G. (1963) *The Concept of the Mind.* London: Penguin.

Riehl J.P. (1974) The Riehl interactional model. In Riehl J.P. & Roy C. (eds) *Conceptual Models in Nursing Practice.* New York: Appleton-Century-Crofts.

Riehl J.P. & Roy C. (1974, 1980) *Conceptual Models in Nursing Practice.* New York: Appleton-Century-Crofts.

Rogers M.E. (1970) *An Introduction to a Theoretical Basis of Nursing*, 1st edition. Philadelphia, PA: F.A. Davis.

Rogers M.E. (1980) *An Introduction to a Theoretical Basis of Nursing*, 2nd edition. Philadelphia: F.A. Davis.

Rolfe G. (1996) *Closing the Theory Practice Gap: A New Paradigm for Nursing.* Oxford, UK: Butterworth Heinemann.

Roper N., Logan N. & Tierney A. (1980, 1985, 1990) *Elements of Nursing*, 1st, 2nd & 3rd editions. Edinburgh, UK: Churchill Livingstone.

Roper N., Logan N. & Tierney A. (1983) *Using a Model for Nursing.* Edinburgh, UK: Churchill-Livingstone.

Roper N., Logan N. & Tierney A.J. (2000) *The Roper-Logan-Tierney Model of Nursing Based on Activities of Living.* Edinburgh, UK: Churchill-Livingstone.

Rose K., Waterman H. & Tullo A. (1997) The extended role of the nurse: reviewing the implications for practice. *Clinical Effectiveness in Nursing*, **1**, 31–37.

Rosenbaum J.N. (1986) Comparison of two theorists on care: Orem and Leininger. *Journal of Advanced Nursing*, **11**, 409–419.

Roy C. (1970) Adaptation: a conceptual framework for nursing. *Nursing Outlook*, **18**(3), 42–45.

Roy C. (1971) Adaptation: a basis for nursing practice. *Nursing Outlook*, **19**(4), 254–257.

Roy C. (1980) The Roy adaptation model. In Riehl J.P. & Roy C. (eds) *Conceptual Models in Nursing Practice.* New York: Appleton-Century-Crofts.

Roy C. (1989) Nursing care in theory and practice: early interventions in brain injury. In Harris R., Burns R. & Rees R. (eds) *Recovery from Brain Injury.* Adelaide, Australia: Institute for the Study of Learning Difficulties.

Roy C. (1999) *Roy Adaptation Model-Based Research: 25 Years of Contributions to Nursing Science.* Indianapolis, IN: Center Nursing Press; Boston Based Adaptation Research in Nursing Society.

Roy C. (2003) Reflections on nursing research and the Roy adaptation model. *Igaju-syoin Japanese Journal*, **36**(1), 7–11.

Ruland C.M. & Moore S.M. (1998) Theory construction based on standards of care: a proposed theory of the peaceful end of life. *Nursing Outlook*, **46**, 169–175.

Ryle G. (1949) *The Concept of Mind.* Chicago: Chicago University Press.

Sackett D.L., Straus S.E., Richardson W.S., Rosenberg W. & Haynes B. (2000) *Evidence-Based Medicine: How to Practice and Teach EBM.* Edinburgh, UK: Churchill Livingstone.

Salanders L. & Dietz-Omar M. (1991) Making nursing models relevant for the practising nurse. *Nursing Practice,* **4**(2), 23–25.

Scholes J. & Vaughan B. (2002) Cross-boundary working: implications for the multiprofessional team. *Journal of Clinical Nursing,* **11**, 399–408.

Scholes J., Furlong S. & Vaughan B. (1999) New roles in practice: charting three typologies of role innovation. *Nursing in Critical Care,* **4**(6), 268–275.

Schön D. (1987) *Educating the Reflective Practitioner.* San Francisco, CA: Jossey Bass.

Semple M. & Cable S. (2003) The new Code of Professional Conduct. *Nursing Standard,* **17**(23), 10–48.

Silva M.C. (1977) Philosophy, science, theory: interrelationships and implications for nursing research. *Image,* **9**(3), 59–63.

Silva M.C., Sorrel J.M. & Sorrel C.D. (1995) From Carper's patterns of knowing to ways of being: an ontological philosophical shift in nursing. *Advances in Nursing Science,* **18**(1), 1–13.

Shelley M. (1996/1831) *Frankenstein, or the Modern Prometheus.* London: W.W. Norton.

Slevin O. (1995) Theories and models. In Bashford P. & Slevin O. (eds) *Theory and Practice in Nursing.* Edinburgh, UK: Campion Press.

Slevin O. (1999) The nurse-patient relationship: caring in a health context. In Long A. (ed.) *Interaction for Practice in Community Nursing.* London: Macmillan.

Slevin O. (2003a) Nursing models and theories: major contributions. In Basford L. & Slevin O. (eds) *Theory and Practice of Nursing: An Integrated Approach to Caring Practice,* 2nd edition. Cheltenham, UK: Nelson Thornes.

Slevin O. (2003b) Nursing as a profession. In Basford L. & Slevin O. (eds) *Theory and Practice of Nursing: An Integrated Approach to Caring Practice,* 2nd edition. Cheltenham, UK: Nelson Thornes.

Slevin O. (2003c) Theory, practice and research. In Basford L. & Slevin O. (eds) *Theory and Practice of Nursing: An Integrated Approach to Caring Practice,* 2nd edition. Cheltenham, UK: Nelson Thornes.

Slevin O. & Kirby C. (2003) Personal knowing: nursing as a caring and healing process. In Basford L. & Slevin O. (eds) *Theory and Practice of Nursing: An Integrated Approach to Caring Practice,* 2nd edition. Cheltenham, UK: Nelson Thornes.

Smith L. (1982) Models of nursing as the basis for curriculum development: some rationales and implications. *Journal of Advanced Nursing,* **7**, 117–127.

Smith L. (1986) Issues raised by the use of nursing models in psychiatry. *Nurse Education Today,* **6**, 69–75.

Smith M.C. (1994) Arriving at a philosophy of nursing: discovering? constructing? evolving? In Kikuchi J.F. & Simmons H. (eds) *Developing a Philosophy of Nursing.* Newbury Park, CA: Sage.

SODH (Scottish Office Department of Health) (1995) *Health Service Developments and The Scope of Professional Nursing Practice: a survey of developing clinical roles within NHS Trusts in Scotland*. National Nursing, Midwifery and Health Visiting Advisory Committee.

Stevens B.J. (1979) *Nursing Theory: Analysis, Application, Evaluation*. Boston, MA: Little, Brown.

Stevens Barnum B.J. (1998) *Nursing Theory: Analysis, Application, Evaluation*. New York: Lippincott Williams & Wilkins.

Stevenson R.L. (2000/1886) *The Strange Case of Dr Jekyll and Mr Hyde*. New York: Bartleby.

Stockwell F. (1985) *The Nursing Process in Psychiatric Nursing*. London: Croom Helm.

Stokes P. (2004) *Philosophy: 100 Essential Thinkers*. London: Capella.

Strauss A. & Corbin J. (1998) *Basics of Qualitative Research: Techniques and Procedures for Developing Grounded Theory*, 2nd edition. Thousand Oaks, CA: Sage.

Sudnow D. (2001) *Ways of the Hand: A Rewritten Account*. Cambridge, MA: MIT Press.

Sullivan H.S. (1953) *The Interpersonal Theory of Psychiatry*. In Perry H.S. & Gawel M.L. (eds). New York: W.W. Norton & Co. Inc.

Suppe F. & Jacox A. (1985) Philosophy of science and the development of nursing theory. In Werley H. & Fitzpatrick J.J. (eds) *Annual Review of Nursing Research*, **3**, 241–267.

Swanson K.M. (1991) Empirical development of a mid range theory of caring. *Nursing Research*, **40**, 241–267.

Taylor C. (1995) *Philosophical Arguments*. Cambridge: MA: Harvard University Press.

Thomas B.J. & Biddle E.J. (1966) Basic concepts for classifying the phenomena of role. In Biddle B.J. & Thomas E.J. (eds) *Role Theory: Concepts and Research*. New York: John Wiley & Sons Inc.

Toulmin S. (1972) *Human Understanding*. Princeton, NJ: Princeton University Press.

Travelbee J. (1966) *Interpersonal Aspects of Nursing*. Philadelphia, PA: F.A. Davis.

UKCC (United Kingdom Central Council for Nursing, Midwifery and Health Visiting) (1992) *The Scope of Professional Practice*. London: UKCC.

UKCC (United Kingdom Central Council for Nursing, Midwifery and Health Visiting) (1999) *Fitness for Practice*. London: UKCC.

UKCC (United Kingdom Central Council for Nursing, Midwifery and Health Visiting) (2002) Report of the higher level of practice pilot and project: Executive Summary. London: UKCC.

Van Manen M. (1999) The pathic nature of inquiry and nursing. In Madjar I. & Walton J. (eds) *Nursing and the Experience of Illness: Phenomenology in Practice*. New York: Routledge.

Von Bertalanffy L. (1951) General systems theory: a new approach to unity of science. *Human Biology*, December, 303–361.

Wachowski L. & Wachowski A. (1999) *The Matrix*. Warner Bros, http://en.wikipedia.org/wiki/The_Matrix.

Wald F.S. & Leonard R.C. (1964) Towards the development of nursing practice theory. *Nursing Research*, **13**(4), 309–313.

Walker L.O. & Avant K.C. (1995) *Strategies for Theory Construction in Nursing*, 3rd edition. New York: Appleton-Century-Crofts.

Walker L.O. & Avant K.C. (2005) *Strategies for Theory Construction in Nursing*, 4th edition. Upper Saddle River, NJ: Pearson Prentice Hall.

Walsh M. (1991) *Models in Clinical Nursing: The Way Forward*. London: Balliere Tindall.

Watson J. (1973, 1979) *A Model of Caring: An Alternative Health Care Model for Nursing Practice and Research*. American Nurses Association.

Watson J. (1985) *Nursing: Human Science and Care*. New York: Appleton-Century-Crofts.

Webb C. (ed.) (1986) *Using Nursing Models Series: Women's Health, Midwifery and Gynaecological Nursing*. London: Hodder & Stoughton.

Weiss C. (1972) *Evaluation Research: Methods of Assessing Program Effectiveness*. Englewood Cliffs, NJ: Prentice Hall.

Weiss C. (1998) *Evaluation: Methods for Studying Programs and Policies*, 2nd edition. Upper Saddle River, NJ: Prentice Hall.

Whall A. (1989) The influence of logical positivism on nursing practice. *Image: Journal of Nurse Scholarship*, **21**, 243–245.

Wiedenbach E. (1964) *Clinical Nursing: A Helping Art*. New York: Springer.

WIHSC (Welsh Institute for Health and Social Care) (2004) *Innovation and Protection: A Framework for Post-Registration Nursing*. Pontypridd, Wales: WIHSC.

Williams C.A. (1979) The nature and development of conceptual frameworks. In Downs F.S. & Fleming J.W. (eds) *Issues in Nursing Research*, pp. 89–106. New York: Appleton-Century-Crofts.

Williams R. (1983) *Keywords*. 2nd edition. London: Fontana.

Wilson A., Averis A. & Walsh K. (2003) The influences on and experiences of becoming nurse entrepreneurs: a Delphi study. *International Journal of Nursing Practice*, **9**, 236–245.

Wimpenny P. (2002) The meaning of models of nursing to practising nurses. *Journal of Advanced Nursing*, **40**(3), 346–354.

Wooldridge P.J. (1992) The author comments. In Nicholl L.H. (ed.) *Perspectives on Nursing Theory*, 2nd edition. Philadelphia, PA: J.B. Lippincott.

Wright S.G. (1985) It's all right in theory. *Nursing Times*, **81**(34), 19–20.

Wright S.G. (1986) *Building and Using a Model of Nursing*. London: Edward Arnold.

Yoo K.H. (1991) Expectation and evaluation of occupational health nursing services, as perceived by occupational health nurses, employees and employers in the United Kingdom. University of Ulster, Unpublished PhD thesis.

Young A., Taylor S.G. & Renpenning K. (2001) *Connections: Nursing Research, Theory and Practice*. St Louis: Mosby, Inc.

Yura H. & Torres G. (1975) Today's conceptual frameworks within Baccalaureate Nursing Programs. In *Faculty-Curriculum Development. Part III. Conceptual Framework, its Meaning and Function*. pp. 17–25. New York: National League of Nursing.

Index

a priori knowing, 42, 77
a priori reasoning, 65
absolute truth, 43
abstract theory
  levels, 44–5
  and reality, 47–9
  see also propositional knowledge
adapted theories, 144–5
advanced nurses
  training issues, 95
  see also nursing roles
aesthetics and knowing, 79–80, 216
Americanisation concerns, 25–6, 119, 149
assumptions, 27
attitudes to theory use, 148

behavioural paradigms, 115–16
Benner, Patricia, 12, 76
'body of knowledge', 7, 11, 16–17

caring, definitions and forms, 127–8
Carper, Barbara, 79–81, 178, 216
Cartesian theories, 26–8, 65–6
'clinical wisdom' (Benner), 12
complexity, and practical knowledge, 35–9
Comte, Auguste, 67–8
concepts, 4–5, 29
  development, 178–82
  labelling, 181
conceptualisations, 109–11
criteria for selecting theories, 149–53
critical science, 73–4

deductive reasoning, 65, 85–6, 163
defeasibility, 43, 187
Descartes, René, 65–6, 85
descriptive theories, 29–30, 176, 177
developmental paradigms, 115
Dickoff, James and James, Patricia, 29–32, 82, 175–6
Diers, Donna, 175–6
Dilthey, Wilhelm, 83–4
documentation issues, 119

empathy, 41
empirical indicators, 44–5
empiricism, 66–70, 163
  and knowing, 79, 215–16
enlightenment, emancipation and empowerment, 74
ethical principles, 50
ethics
  and knowing, 80
  and science, 49–52
  and theory selection, 143–4
ethnography, 165
evaluation of nursing theories, 173–5, 185–217
  differentiation, 198
  dimensions, 187, 198, 204, 210, 213
  frameworks, 211–15
  key approaches, 202–7
  models, 203
  terminology and language, 186–8
    'evaluation and worth', 190–92
    'quality', 195–6
    'right and wrong', 189–90
    'standards and quality', 192–5
    'value and theory', 196–8
  testing, 198–202
  through research, 204–7
  use of summative and formative methods, 207–10
evidence-based nursing, and theory, 11–12, 31–2
explanatory theories, 29–30, 176–7
explicit knowing, 76
extended nursing roles, 91–2

falsification testing, 69
Fawcett, J., 214
formative evaluation, 207–9
fragmentation of the person, 13–14, 15
frameworks, 17
  for evaluation, 211–15
  for research, role of theories, 171–3
  see also paradigms
Frankfurt School, 73–4
Freud, Sigmund, 65

Galilei, Galileo (1564–1642), 7, 70
global risk, 54
gnostic touch, 40
grand theories, 44–5
    relevance to nursing, 100–102, 142–3
grounded theory, 24–5, 165
growth and development *see* developmental
        paradigms
'gut reaction' *see* tacit knowledge (Polanyi)

health, metaparadigm components, 118
Heidegger, Martin, 72–3
hermeneutics, 73
hierarchy of evidence, 78
historicism, 70–71
holistic care, theories and concepts, 13–14, 15
home-grown theories, 156–7
hospital stays, 147
human science, and research, 83–4
human state, 27–8
Husserl, Edmund, 72
hypotheses, 44
hypotheses-testing studies, 163
    situation-producing theories, 19, 32, 82–3, 163
    see also deductive reasoning; research

imported theories, 25–6, 119, 149
inductive reasoning, 85
information sources, web addresses, 158
'intelligent nursing', 12
interactional paradigm, 114–15
interpersonal relationships and social capital,
        135–6
interpersonal relationships and theory,
        125–39
    descriptions from nursing care, 126–7
    key theory developments, 128–31
        Peplau's theory, 132–4
    threats and challenges, 136–8
        pace of modern healthcare, 136–7
        performance measurement issues, 137
        role drift, 138
        technological developments, 137–8
interpersonal theories, 128–31
    Peplau's theory, 132–4
    threats and challenges, 136–8
interprofessional care coordinator roles, 93–4
interprofessional working, 92–3
intuition, 146
    and scientific empiricism, 69
    see also tacit knowledge (Polanyi)
isolation, 125–6

jargon issues, 119–20, 152
justified knowledge, 43

Kerlinger, F.N.B., 77–8
King, Imogen, 129–31
'know-how' notions, 34–5, 36, 58–9, 75–6
'know-that' notions, 75–6
'know-why' notions, 76
knowing
    categories, 77–8
    different types, 47
    in nursing, 75–6
        Carper's four patterns, 79–81, 178, 216
        patterns and taxonomy, 16, 216
knowing and theory, 82–3, 215–16

knowledge
    definitions, 63–4
    nature and types, 34–45
        practical knowledge, 8–9, 30, 33–4, 34–41
        propositional knowledge, 33–4, 41–5
    philosophical views on development, 64–71
        empiricism, 66–70
        historicism, 70–71
        phenomenology, 72–3
        rationalism, 64–6
        of science, 71–2
        theory–model conceptualisations, 110–11
knowledge building, 30
knowledge confirming, 30
knowledge utilisation, 30
Kuhn, Thomas, 71

language use *see* terminology issues
Laudan, Larry, 71–2
levels of theory, 29–32, 82, 96, 100–104
    and abstract entities, 44–5
    and levels of research, 175–6
Locke, John, 67
logical positivism, 69–70

McKenna, H.P., 142, 174–5, 214
McKenna, H.P. and Slevin, O.D., 214
macro theory *see* grand theories
market forces, 51–2
medical models
    influence on nursing roles, 96–100
    political and social pressures, 146
Meleis, A.I., 178–82
Merton, Thomas, 21–3, 57–8
metaparadigm, 116–18
metatheory, 28, 45
micro theory *see* practice theories
middle range theories, 44
    examples, 143
    relevance to nursing, 102–3, 142–3
midwifery nursing theories, 149
mind–body split, 66
models, 107–9
    descriptions, 107–8
    dimensional formats, 108–9
    as precursor of theory, 110
morality and science, 49–52
Muir Gray, J.A., 78
multidisciplinary theories, 156–7
multiple theory use, 146–7

neo-modernity *see* post modernity
Nightingale, Florence, 74, 96–7
non-registered nursing staff, 93
nurse specialists, 93–4
    and deskilling of general practitioners, 95–6
nurse training *see* training and education
nurses, as metatheorists, 28
nursing knowledge
    development theories, 71–2, 74–6
    development through reasoning, 85–7
    know-how/-that/-why, 75–6
    metaparadigm components, 118
    patterns of knowing, 79–81
    see also knowing; knowledge
nursing roles
    concepts and theories, 90–92
    extension and expansion changes, 91–2

causing confusion, 93–4
deskilling of general practitioners, 95–6
inconsistencies, 95
into medical roles, 98–100
isolation and burnout concerns, 94–5
responsibility and accountability issues, 94
influences of medical model, 96–100
interprofessional changes, 92–3
relevance of different theory levels, 96, 100–104
nursing science, 54
development theories, 71–2
nursing theories, 128–9
categories, 129
early 'grand' theories, 129–31
Peplau's theory, 132–4
evaluations, 173–5
evolution and development strategies, 178–83
implications for education, 134–5
number of different entities, 142
selection considerations, 141–57
challenges and problems, 143–9
criteria, 149–53
strategies, 154–7
use of paradigms, 153
use of staff values and beliefs, 153–4
threats to interpersonal approaches, 136–8
use of home-grown theories, 156–7
web addresses, 158
see also theory in nursing
nursing theorists, 129–31

objective truth, and positivism, 69
Orem's self-care theory, 112, 143
Orlando, Ida, 129–31
outcome evaluations see evaluation of nursing
theories; performance measurement
ownership of theories, 156–7

paradigms, 13, 17
and nursing theories, 114–15, 153
pathic touch, 40–41
Peplau's theory, 132–4
key assumptions, 132–3
phases and roles, 133
performance measurement, 137
personal knowing, 35, 80–81
phenomena, 160
phenomenology, 72–4, 165
Polanyi, Michael, 14, 35, 38, 76
Popper, Karl, 43, 55, 66, 69, 160–61
positivism, 53, 163
early developments and origins, 68–9
post modernity, 56–7
post-positivism, 55–7
post-positivist empiricism, 69–70
postmodernism, 55–7
practical knowledge, 34–41
as performance, 39
as sophisticated knowledge, 39–41
and theory, 8–9, 30, 33–4
see also practice
practice
concepts, 23–4
and nursing theory, 8–9, 23–5, 33–4
informing and guiding theory, 19, 24–5, 159–68
and research, 159–64
practice theories, 44
relevance to nursing, 103–4

praxis, 1, 19, 46
predictive theories, 29–31, 177–8
prescriptive theory, 29–31
propositional diagramming, 167–8
see also propositions
propositional knowledge, 41–5
and justified knowledge, 43
levels, 44–5
and rational knowing, 41–2
as theory, 44–5
vs. practical knowledge, 33–4
see also propositions; theory in nursing; theory-
generating research (TGR)
propositions, 4–5, 29
definitions, 42
development, 181–2

qualitative research, 84, 160–63
quality standards see 'standards and quality'
quantitative research, 84

randomised controlled trials (RCTs), 78
rational knowing, 41–2
see also propositional knowledge
rationalism, 64–6
reality
and abstract theories, 48–9
and science, 47–9
reasoning
and development of nursing knowledge,
85–7
types, 85–7
reflection during practice, 39
reflexive modernity see post modernity
reflexivity, 57
Reid, Trish, 160–61, 163
relationships see interpersonal relationships and
theory
research
concepts, 7–8
definitions, 83
and knowledge development, 83–5
moral and ethical considerations, 49–51
and theory, 159–83
empirical relationships, 175–8
evaluating theories, 173–5
four key links, 163–4
framing of theories, 171–3
generation and development of theories,
164–8
strategies for theory development, 178–83
testing of theories, 168–71
see also science and theory
research governance, 50–51
retroductive reasoning, 86
'right and wrong', 189–90
risk society, 53–4
role conflict, 91
role confusion, 92, 93
role drift, 138
role expansion and extension, 91–2
see also nursing roles
role theory, 90–92
Ryle, Gilbert, 36

science and knowledge development, 71–2, 188
see also research
science and reality, 47–9

science and theory, 7–8, 12, 18–19, 49–54
    disappointing the world, 53–4
    divorced from real world concerns, 49–51
    failing or saving the world, 51–2
    moral and ethical responsibilities, 49–52
    see also nursing science; research
science–practice gap, 47–57
    real world concerns, 47–9
        moral and ethical responsibilities, 49–52
        risk issues, 53–4
    see also technological developments
scientism, 52
selection of theories see theory selection
sick roles, 98
Silva, Mary, 146
situation-producing theories, 19, 32, 82–3, 163
skills, 39–40
    see also practical knowledge
social capital, 135–6
social relationships see interpersonal relationships
        and theory
'standards and quality', 192–5
Sudnow, David, 36–7, 40
summative evaluation, 207–9
sympathy, 41
systems, concepts and descriptions, 114
systems paradigm, 114

tacit knowledge (Polanyi), 14, 35, 76, 146
    see also practical knowledge
technological developments, 137–8
terminology issues, 119–20, 152
    and evaluation, 186–8
        'evaluation and worth', 190–92
        'quality', 195–6
        'right and wrong', 189–90
        'standards and quality', 192–5
        'value and theory', 196–7
testing nursing theories, 198–202
    see also evaluation of nursing theories
theoretical frameworks, 171–3
theorising, defined, 27
theory
    classification systems, 113–16
        behavioural paradigm, 115
        developmental paradigm, 115
        interactional paradigm, 114–15
        systems paradigm, 114
        and metaparadigms, 116–18
    definitions and conceptualisations, 109–11, 129
    development and evolution aspects, 112–13
        strategies, 178–83
    evaluation and testing, 198–217
    model precursors, 110–11
theory in nursing
    aims and rationale for use, 1–3, 10–12, 19
    benefits, 122–4
    critiques and limitations, 13–15, 25–6, 46–7,
        119–21
    definitions, 3–5, 6, 10
        reflections, 6–9, 18–19
    development and evolution, 112–13
        strategies, 178–83
    evaluation and testing, 173–5, 198–217
        terminology issues, 186–98
    key elements (Popper), 18–19
    levels and uses, 29–32, 82, 96
        entities or types, 44–5, 100–104
        relevance to nursing, 96, 100–104

relationship to nursing practice, 8–9, 23–5, 58–60,
        96
    and knowing, 82–3
    and situation-producing theories, 19, 32, 82–3
relevance for nurses, 26, 32, 100–104
    concept critiques, 121
    'the theory–practice gap', 8, 46–7, 121
selection considerations, 141–57
    challenges and problems, 143–9
    criteria, 149–53
wider contexts, 16–17
    see also interpersonal theories
theory and relationships see interpersonal
        relationships and theory
theory and research, 159–83
    empirical relationships, 175–8
    evaluating theories, 173–5
    framing of theories, 171–3
    generation and development of theories,
        164–8
    strategies for theory development, 178–83
    testing of theories, 168–71
theory selection
    criteria, 149–53
    key challenges, 143–9
        inappropriate choices, 148
        levels of knowledge, 145
        restrictiveness issues, 147–8
        social and political influences, 145–6
        staff attitudes, 148
        time constraints, 147
        use of merged or adapted theories, 144–5
        use of multiple theories, 146–7
    strategies, 154?
    use of paradigms, 153
    use of practitioner beliefs and values, 153–4
'the theory–practice gap', 8, 46–7, 121
theory-evaluating research (TER), 173–5
theory-framed research (TFR), 171–3
theory-generating research (TGR), 164–8
    key approaches, 165–6
    processes, 166–8
    relationship with TTR, 171
theory-of-action, 19
    see also situation-producing theories
theory-testing research (TTR), 168–71
    processes, 169–71
    relationship with TGR, 171
thinking, 26–7
time constraints, 136–7
    length of patient stay, 147
training and education, influence of nursing
        theories, 134–5
Travelbee, Joyce, 129–31
truth, 43
    and intuition, 146
    and postmodernism, 55–7
    and theory, 145
    through rigorous research, 77

values and beliefs, influence on choice of theory,
        153–4
van Manen, Max, 40
Vienna Circle, 69

Walker, L.O. and Avant, K.C., 214
worldviews, 13–14, 113
    see also paradigms
'worth', 190–92